SSSHHH!!! THE BURIAL

Christ Consciousness
Checks
&
Balances

Chase Duquesnay
Dr. EnQi ReaL

Amazon

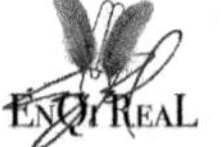

ISBN: 9798302667311

Cover design by: EnQi ReaL

Printed in the United States of America

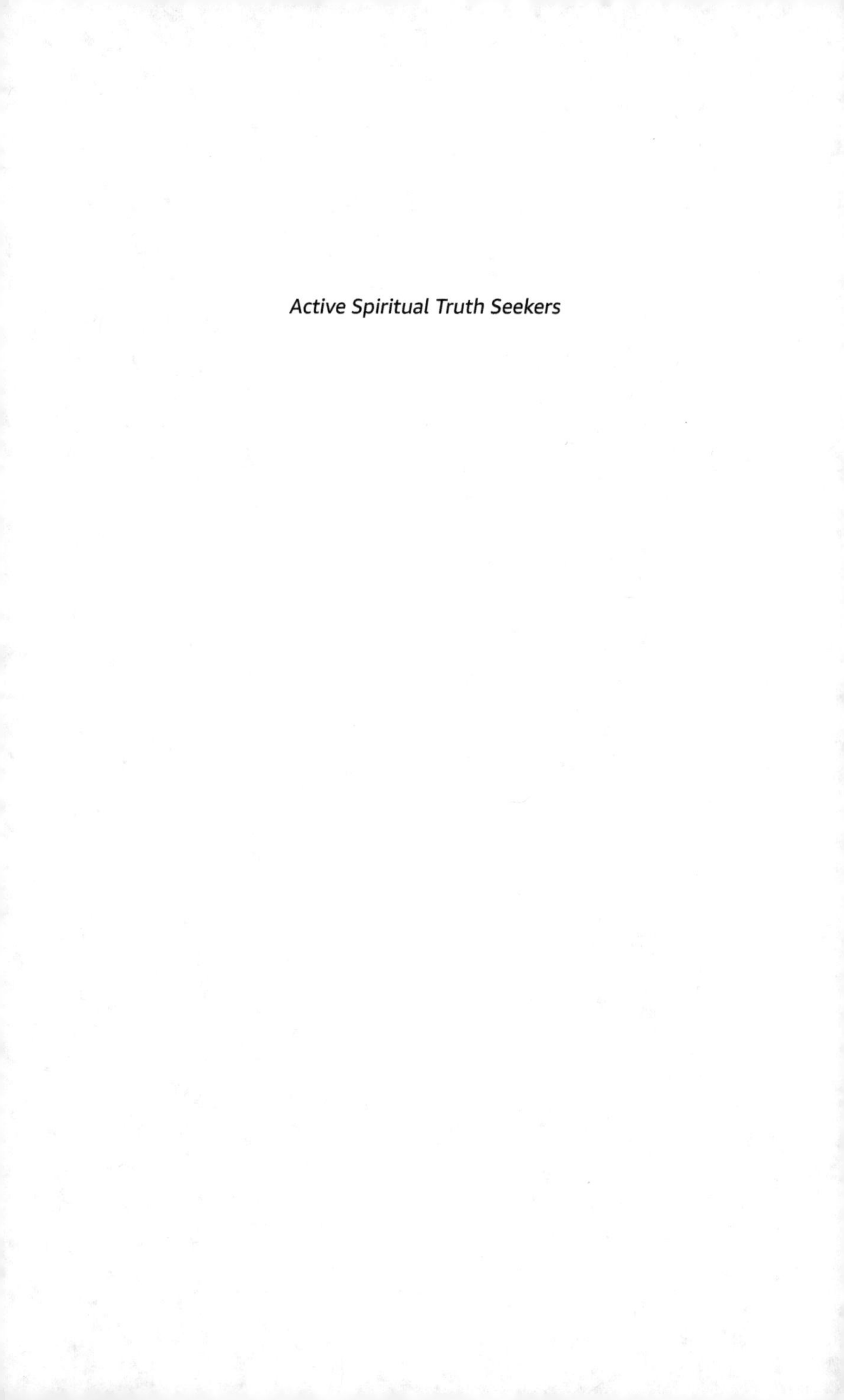
Active Spiritual Truth Seekers

CONTENTS

INTRODUCTION

You can not be a Jewish, Israelite, Christian, Muslim or any other Monotheistic practicing person, and also deal with Chakras. Leave that alone unless you are a Buddhist and you are studying the Upanishads.

This is book is more Prayer... for the Electricians. You should always pray facing the Great Pyramid! I am a Kemetic Student and a Christian (Nazarene).

CHRIST

English is a Magical Language. English is not from England. English is 52% French / 48% German (debatably) and it is written in a Roman version of Hebrew. English has a Alphabet and Hebrew has a AlephBeyt.

P - mouth; sixteenth letter of the English alphabet, descended from the Greek pi; the form of it is a pi with the second limb curved around to meet the first. A rare letter in the initial position in Germanic, in part because by Grimm's Law PIE p- became Germanic f-; even including the early Latin borrowings in Old English, "P" has only a little over 4 pages in J.R. Clark Hall's "Concise Anglo-Saxon Dictionary," compared to 31 pages for B and more than 36 for F. But it now is the third-most-common initial letter in the English vocabulary, and with C and S comprises nearly a third of the dictionary, a testimony to the flood of words that have entered the language since 1066 from Latin, Greek, and French, especially those in pre- and pro-.

Between -m- and another consonant, an

unetymological -p- sometimes is inserted (Hampstead, Thompson) to indicate that the -m- is sounded as in words such as Simpson. To mind one's Ps and Qs (1779), possibly is from confusion of these letters among children learning to write. Another theory traces it to old-time tavern-keepers tracking their patrons' bar tabs in pints and quarts. But see also to be P and Q (1610s), "to be excellent," a slang or provincial phrase said to derive from prime quality. **P-wave is from 1908 in geology, the p representing primary** (adj.). The U.S. Navy World War II PT boat (1942) stands for patrol torpedo.

Q - Back of the Head; 16th letter of the classical Roman alphabet, occurring in English only before a -u- that is followed by another vowel (with a few exceptions; see below), whether the -u- is sounded or not (pique). The letter is from the Phoenician equivalent of Hebrew **koph, qoph**, which was used for the deeper and more guttural of the two "k" sounds in Semitic. The letter existed in early Greek (where there was no such distinction), and called koppa, but it was little used and not alphabetized; it mainly served as a sign of number (90).

The connection with -u- began in Latin. Anglo-Saxon scribes at first adopted the habit, but later used spellings with cw- or cu-. The qu- pattern returned to English with the Normans and French after the

Conquest and had displaced cw- by c. 1300.

In some spelling variants of late Middle English, quh- also took work from wh-, especially in Scottish and northern dialects, for example Gavin Douglas, Provost of St. Giles, in his vernacular "Aeneid" of 1513:
Lyk as the rois in June with hir sueit smell
The marygulde or dasy doith excell.
Quhy suld I than, with dull forhede and vane,
With ruide engine and barrand emptive brane,
With bad harsk speche and lewit barbour tong,
Presume to write quhar thi sueit bell is rong,
Or contirfait sa precious wourdis deir?

Scholars use -q- alone to transliterate Semitic koph or the equivalent in Turkish or Iranian (as in Quran, Qatar, Iraq). In Christian theology, Q has been used since 1901 to signify the hypothetical source of passages shared by Matthew and Luke but not in Mark; in this sense probably it is an abbreviation of German Quelle "source" (from Old High German quella, from the same Proto-Germanic source as Old English cwiella, cwylla "spring; well"). In Middle English accounts, it is an abbreviation of quadrans "farthing" (mid-15c.). In Roman personal names it is an abbreviation of Quintus.

R - **Resh/Head**; eighteenth letter of the English alphabet, traceable to Phoenician and always representing more or less the same sound, which in many languages is typically so resonant and continuous as to be nearly akin to the vowels, but in English is closer to -l-.

It was aspirated at the start of words (hr-) in Old English, as in Greek, but this was abandoned in English spelling and pronunciation by the end of the Old English period, but the rh- spelling survives in many words borrowed from Greek. In many languages and some dialects (e.g. Scottish) it is pronounced with a distinct trilling vibration of the tongue-tip, which gave it its ancient nickname of "the dog letter;" in other regional dialects (e.g. Boston) it is omitted unless followed by a vowel, while in others it is introduced artificially in pronunciation ("idear," "drawring," tomorrer for tomorrow is attested in print by 1901).

If all our r's that are written are pronounced, the sound is more common than any other in English utterance (over seven per cent.); the instances of occurrence before a vowel, and so of universal pronunciation, are only half as frequent. There are localities where the normal vibration of the tip of the tongue is replaced by one of the uvula, making a guttural trill, which is still more entitled to the name of "dog's letter" than is the ordinary r; such are considerable parts of France and Germany; the sound appears to occur only sporadically in English pronunciation. [Century Dictionary]

Louise Pound ("The Humorous 'R'") notes that in British humorous writing, -ar- "popularly indicates the sound of the vowel in father" and formations like larf (for laugh) "are to be read with the broad vowel but no uttered r."

The moment we encounter the added r's of purp or dorg in our reading we know that we have to do with humor, and so with school-marm. The added consonants are supposed to be spoken, if the words are uttered, but, as a matter of fact, they are less often uttered than seen. The words are, indeed, largely visual forms; the humor is chiefly for the eye. [Louise Pound, "The Humorous 'R,'" American Mercury, October 1924]
H.A. Shands ("Some Peculiarities of Speech in Mississippi," 1893) notes uh as "The common negro form for the indefinite article a," and adds, "This is generally written er by dialect writers but no sound of r is ever apparent in the negro pronunciation."
Louise Pound also quotes Henry James on the characteristic prominence of the medial -r- sound (which tends to be dropped in England and New England) in the speech of the U.S. Midwest, "under some strange impulse received toward consonantal recovery of balance, making it present even in words from which it is absent, bringing it in everywhere as with the small vulgar effect of a sort of morose grinding of the back teeth."

In a circle, meaning "registered (trademark),"

attested by 1925. R&R "rest and relaxation," is attested by 1953, American English; R&B "rhythm and blues" (type of popular music) is attested by 1949, American English. Form three Rs, see Three Rs.

S - S, or for lowercase, s, is the nineteenth letter of the Latin alphabet, used in the English alphabet, the alphabets of other western European languages and other latin alphabets worldwide. Its name in English is ess[a] (pronounced /ˈɛs/), plural esses. Northwest Semitic šîn represented a voiceless postalveolar fricative /ʃ/ (as in 'ship'). It originated most likely as a pictogram of a tooth (שׁנא) and represented the phoneme /ʃ/ via the acrophonic principle.

Ancient Greek did not have a /ʃ/ "sh" phoneme, so the derived Greek letter Sigma (Σ) came to represent the voiceless alveolar sibilant /s/. While the letter shape Σ continues **Phoenician šîn**, its name sigma is taken from the letter Samekh, while the shape and position of samekh but name of šîn is continued in the xi.[citation needed] Within Greek, the name of sigma was influenced by its association with the Greek word σίζω (earlier *sigj-), "to hiss". The original name of the letter "Sigma" may have been san, but due to the early history of the Greek epichoric alphabets, "san" came to be identified as a separate letter, Ϻ.

 Herodotus reported that "san" was the name given by the Dorians to the same letter called "Sigma" by the Ionians.

The Western Greek alphabet used in Cumae was adopted by the Etruscans and Latins in the 7th century BC, and over the following centuries, it developed into a range of Old Italic alphabets, including the Etruscan alphabet and the early Latin alphabet. In Etruscan, the value /s/ of Greek sigma (□) was maintained, while san (□) represented a separate phoneme, most likely /ʃ/ "sh" (transliterated as ś). The early Latin alphabet adopted sigma, but not san, as Old Latin did not have a /ʃ/ "sh" phoneme.

The shape of Latin S arises from Greek Σ by dropping one out of the four strokes of that letter. The (angular) S-shape composed of three strokes existed as a variant of the four-stroke letter Σ already in the epigraphy of Western Greek alphabets, and the three and four strokes variants existed alongside one another in the classical Etruscan alphabet. In other Italic alphabets (Venetic, Lepontic), the letter could be represented as a zig-zagging line of any number between three and six strokes. The Italic letter was also adopted into Elder Futhark, as Sowilō (ᛊ), and appears with four to eight strokes in the earliest runic inscriptions, but is occasionally reduced to three strokes (ᛋ) from the later 5th century, and appears regularly with three strokes in Younger Futhark.

The ⟨sh⟩ digraph for English /ʃ/ arose in Middle

English (alongside ⟨sch⟩), replacing the Old English ⟨sc⟩ digraph. Similarly, Old High German ⟨sc⟩ was replaced by ⟨sch⟩ in Early Modern High German orthography.

In English, ⟨s⟩ represents a voiceless alveolar sibilant /s/. It also commonly represents a voiced alveolar sibilant /z/, as in 'rose' and 'bands'. Due to yod-coalescence, it may also represent a voiceless palato-alveolar fricative /ʃ/, as in 'sugar', or a voiced palato-alveolar fricative /ʒ/, as in 'measure'.

Final ⟨s⟩ is the usual mark for plural nouns. It is the regular ending of English third person present tense verbs.

In some words of French origin, ⟨s⟩ is silent, as in 'isle' or 'debris'.

The letter ⟨s⟩ is the seventh most common letter in English and the third-most common consonant after ⟨t⟩ and ⟨n⟩. It is the most common letter for the first letter of a word in the English language.

T - Tau/Nilometer; twentieth letter of the English alphabet; in the Phoenician alphabet the corresponding sign was the 22nd and last; all beyond T in the modern alphabet represents European alterations or additions. The sound has been consistent throughout its history. The letter formerly was branded on the hand of a convicted thief. Also compare th.

In Late Latin and Old French, -t- before -e- and -iacquired the "s" value of -c- and words appeared in both spellings (nationem/nacionem) and often passed into Middle English with a -c- (nacioun). In most of these the spelling was restored to a -t- by or during early Modern English. Edmund Coote's "English Schoole-maister" (1596) still has malicious/malitious; and a few words well-established in the old spelling (space, place, coercion, suspicion) resisted restoration.

The pronunciation shift in -tu- words in southern English, to "-shu-" (nature, actually), was noticed by c. 1900.

To cross one's t's (and dot one's i's) "be exact" is attested from 1849. Phrase to a T "exactly, with utmost exactness" is recorded from 1690s, though the exact signification remains uncertain despite much speculation. The measuring tool called a T-square (sometimes suggested as the source of this) is recorded by that name only from 1785.
In medicine, the T-cell (1970) is so called because the cells are derived from the thymus. As a medieval numeral, T represented 160.

QRST (Breakdown by letters) - Back of the Head, Apis (Final), Front of the Head, Flag (Most High, Most Important), Shin, 3 Flags (Destroy, Consume), Tau, Nilometer, 19 (Cross, Covenant, Seal)!!!

YaShua
YahShua

YahoShua
Joshua son of Nun (Fish)

We know that Jesus is not the 'real' thing. Jesus is a derivative of Zeus.

We are dealing with the Christ part! I think this is very important, we know where Hebrew comes from. Christ refers specifically to Osiris, not a random Messenger or one who is Anointed.

Christ - The word is derived from the Greek verb χρίω (chrī̄ō), meaning literally "to anoint." In the Greek Septuagint, χριστός was a semantic loan used to translate the Hebrew מָשִׁיחַ (Mašíaḥ, messiah), meaning "[one who is] anointed". There is more to this word Christ and its related Hebrew word Messiah. Messiah is not a translation but a transliteration of the Hebrew word mashiach. The root of מָשִׁיחַ is מ-שׁ-ח which means "anoint" or "'measure".

Listen we have to put this on wax (pun intended). To rub with Oil? That is literally apart of the Mummification or Embalming process. We know the 'Djews' got this from Kemet as per the Burials we see in the Bible. The thing is Christ in the Bible rose! Being raised is a reference to Shu, the empty tomb in the cave is a reference to 'Shu's' Chamber in the Pyramid. This is insane, do you see that you are the body of Christ yet?

Osiris was the first King, a man (at least symbolized as one). Shu was the God who Created the Heaven (Nuit) and Earth (Geb). Osiris, Ausar, Wusir represents Man, he pioneered death. He pioneered the Afterlife, the path to the Cross (Scale). The Living God of Light and Life though, is Shu.

Osiris - Buried in your Chest

Chest - Middle English chest, from Old English cest "box, **coffer**, **casket**," usually large and with a hinged lid, from Proto-Germanic *kista (source also of Old Norse and Old High German kista, Old Frisian, Middle Dutch, German kiste, Dutch kist). This is an early borrowing from Latin cista "**chest**, **box**," from Greek kistē "a box, basket," from PIE *kista "woven container" (Beekes compares Middle Irish cess "basket, causeway of wickerwork, bee-hive," Old Welsh cest).

The meaning of the English word was extended to "thorax, **trunk of the body from the neck to the diaphragm**" c. 1400, replacing breast (n.) in that sense, on the **metaphor of the ribs as a "box" for the heart**.

The meaning "place where public money is kept (common chest, mid-15c.) was extended to "public funds" (1580s). Chest of drawers is from 1670s.

The Amduat, Book of Gates, Underworld of Osiris... They are all telling you something, so is modern science. Keep in mind, the same way Hebrew & Arabic come from Mdu Ntr, Modern Science comes from Kemet as well.

In hour 1 the sun god enters the western horizon (akhet) which is a transition between day and night.

In hours 2 and 3 he passes through an abundant watery world called 'Wernes' and the 'Waters of Osiris'.

In hour 4 he reaches the difficult sandy realm of Sokar, the underworld hawk deity, where he encounters dark zig zag pathways which he has to negotiate, being dragged on a snake-boat.

In hour 5 he discovers the tomb of Osiris which is an enclosure beneath which is hidden a lake of fire, the tomb is covered by a pyramid like mound (identified with the goddess Isis) and on top of which Isis and Nephthys have alighted in the form of two kites (birds of prey).

In the sixth hour the most significant event in the underworld occurs. The ba (or soul) of Ra unites with his own body, or alternatively with the ba of Osiris within the circle formed by the mehen serpent. This event is the point at which the sun begins its regeneration, it is a moment of great significance, but also danger, as beyond it in hour 7 the adversary Apep (Apophis) lies in wait and has to be subdued by the magic of Isis, and the strength of Set assisted by

Serqet.

Once this has been done the sun god opens the doors of the tomb in hour 8 and then leaves the sandy island of Sokar by rowing vigorously back into the waters in hour 9.

In hour 10 the regeneration process continues through immersion in the waters until in hour 11 the gods eyes (a symbol for his health and well being) are fully regenerated.

In hour 12 he enters the eastern horizon ready to rise again as the new day's sun.

The Amduat, Book of Gates, Underworld of Osiris... They are all telling you something, so is modern science. Keep in mind, the same way Hebrew & Arabic come from Mdu Ntr, Modern Science comes from Kemet as well.

1st gate: Sia (deification of perception) standing on the prow of the sun boat, invites a snake called "Desert-Protector" to unlock the gate to the arrival of Ra who, in the form of the god Atum (deification of the sunset sun), observes his enemies being massacred.

2nd gate: the guardian god is called "Swallower Of Sinners" and his gate precedes a lake of fire.

3rd gate: its guardian snake is "Stinger" while the portal itself is the goddess "Mistress Of Food"; some jackals watch over the "Lake of Life" interdicted to the dead because it is the place where Ra draws his breath.

4th gate: some deities carry ropes to measure the extension of the netherworld fields — as well as, in the daily life of the Egyptians, the measurement of the fields was carried out for tax purposes; this is also where the four human ethnic groups (according to the Egyptians) were depicted: the "cattle of Ra", i.e. Egyptians themselves, Levantines, Libyans, and Nubians.

5th gate: this gate is the goddess "Lady Of Duration" while its guardian serpent is "Flame-Eyed"; this access is inhabited by the perfidious demon Apep — embodiment of evil and chaos (Isfet), bitter enemy of Ra — here called "Evil Of Face". 20 deities manage to stem his devastating power by continuing to dissect it, while the heads of those he devoured emerge from his coils. The sun boat moves on and Ra leaves this dramatic region.

6th gate: Ra's boat approaches to seven jackal-headed poles with two enemies bound to each one, waiting to be beheaded.

7th gate: this gate is the goddess "Shining One" and beyond it there are 20 gods holding a rope ending in four whips, four falcon heads and four human heads. This is an enigmatic and barely understandable point.

8th gate: this access is inhabited by a flaming snake who burns up the enemies of Osiris.

9th gate: here stand Horus and Set on a hawk-headed lion.

10th gate: Apep appears again, but chained in order not to harm Ra in his transit.

11th gate: this gate is called "Mysterious Of Approaches" and is overseen by the cat-headed god Meeyuty (meow onomatopoeia).

12th gate: here stand the goddesses Isis and Nephthys in the form of snakes: the journey through the gates of the afterlife is finished and the sun rises on the world in the form of a sacred scarab (Khepri, deification of the morning sun).

The Amduat, Book of Gates, Underworld of Osiris... They are all telling you something, so is modern science. Keep in mind, the same way Hebrew & Arabic come from Mdu Ntr, Modern Science comes from Kemet as well.

1. The Hall of Judgment (Maat): The soul is judged by Osiris and the 42 divine judges. The heart of the deceased is weighed against the feather of Maat (truth and justice).

2. The Field of Reeds (Aaru): A paradise where the blessed souls reside, akin to a perfect version of the Nile Delta.

3. The Waters of Chaos (Nun): A primordial watery abyss representing the chaos before creation.

4. The Land of Fire: A place of punishment for the wicked, where souls face various torments.

5. The Lake of Fire: Another area of punishment, often depicted as a lake filled with flames.

6. The Hall of the Two Truths: A court where the deceased's deeds are evaluated.

7. The House of the Dead: A dwelling place for souls awaiting judgment.

8. The Abyss: A dark, chaotic region that some souls may encounter.

9. The Serpent's Domain: A place filled with serpents and other dangers, often associated with threats to the soul.

10. The Fields of Iaru: Similar to the Field of Reeds, this is a realm of peace and abundance for the righteous.

11. The Valley of the Dead: A desolate area where souls wander if they are unworthy.

12. The Duat's Gates: Various gates that the soul must pass through, each guarded by a deity, requiring the recitation of spells for safe passage.

The Amduat, Book of Gates, Underworld of Osiris... They are all telling you something, so is modern science. Keep in mind, the same way Hebrew & Arabic come from Mdu Ntr, Modern Science comes from Kemet as well.

The SouL:

1. The Ba, the personality, character. shown as a bird with the head of the deceased.
2. The Ka, the double. Represented by a pair of raised arms.
3. **The Ib, the heart, the seat of the soul. Serves as a record of good and bad deeds. Used at the scales of justice to determine passage into Aaru, paradise.**
4. The Sheut, the shadow.
5. The Ren, the name. A name (carved, written, painted, spoken, etc.) is required for a soul to make return trips to the mortal world. It also contains their experiences and memories.
6. The Khet, the body. Needs to be preserved as well as possible so that the Ka and Ba can return to it and use it. The "opening of the mouth" existed to reanimate the Khet.
7. The Sah, the spiritual body. (A Ghost?)
8. The Sekhem, the 'form 'or 'power'. (life force?)
9. The Akh, the thought or conciousness. A combination of Ba and Ka.

The Amduat, Book of Gates, Underworld of Osiris...

They are all telling you something, so is modern science. Keep in mind, the same way Hebrew & Arabic come from Mdu Ntr, Modern Science comes from Kemet as well.

Traveling through the Heart:

1 Superior Vena Cava
2 Inferior Vena Cava
3 Right Atrium
4 Tricuspid Valve
5 Right ventricle
6 Pulmonary semilunar valve
7 Right/left pulmonary artery
8 Right/left pulmonary vein
9 Left atrium
10 Mitral/Bicuspid Valve
11 Left ventricle
12 Aortic semilunar valve
*13 Was/Aorta

The Amduat, Book of Gates, Underworld of Osiris... They are all telling you something, so is modern science. Keep in mind, the same way Hebrew & Arabic come from Mdu Ntr, Modern Science comes from Kemet as well.

Cava - cava, from cavus "hollow" (from PIE root *keue- "to swell," also "vault, hole").

Atrium - 1570s, in ancient Roman architecture, **<u>entrance-hall</u>,**" the most important and usually the most splendid apartment of a house. from Latin atrium "central court or first main room of a house, room which contains the hearth," from Proto-Italic *atro-, sometimes said (on authority of Varro, "De Lingua Latina") to be Etruscan.

Watkins suggests it is from PIE root *ater- "fire," on notion of "**place where smoke from the hearth escapes**" (through a hole in the roof). De Vaan finds this not very compelling, "since soot is black, but not the fire itself," and prefers a different PIE root, *hert-r- "fireplace," with cognates in Old Irish aith, Welsh odyn "**furnace, oven**," Avestan atarš "**fire**."

The appurtenance of atrium depends on the interpretation that this room originally contained the fireplace. This etymology was already current in ancient times, but there is no independent evidence for it. Still, there is no good alternative. [de Vaan]

The anatomical sense of "either of the upper cavities of the heart" is recorded by 1870. The meaning "sky-lit central court in a public building" is attested by 1967.

Valve - late 14c., "**one of the halves of a folding door**," from Latin valva (plural valvae) "section of a folding or revolving door," literally "that which turns," related to volvere "to roll," from PIE root *wel-(3) "to turn, **revolve**." Sense extended 1610s to "membranous fold regulating flow of bodily fluids;" 1650s to "**mechanical device that works like an anatomical valve**;" and 1660s in zoology to "halves of a hinged shell." Related: Valved.

Artery - late 14c., "an arterial blood vessel," from Anglo-French arterie, Old French artaire (13c.; Modern French artère), and directly from Latin arteria, from Greek arteria "windpipe," also "an artery," as distinct from a vein; related to aeirein "to raise" (see aorta).

They were **regarded by the ancients as air ducts because the arteries do not contain blood after death**, and 14c.-16c. artery in English also could mean "trachea, windpipe." Medieval writers, based on Galen, generally took them as a separate blood system for the "**vital spirits**." The word is used in reference to artery-like systems of major rivers from 1805; of railways from 1844.

Vein - c. 1300, from Old French veine "vein, artery, pulse" (12c.), from Latin vena "a blood vessel," also "a water course, a vein of metal, a person's natural ability or interest," of unknown origin. The mining sense is attested in English from late 14c. (Greek phleps "vein" had the same secondary sense). Figurative sense of "strain or intermixture" (of some quality) is recorded from 1560s; that of "a humor or mood, natural tendency" is first recorded 1570s.

Ventricle - late 14c., "**small chamber** or cavity within a bodily organ," especially of the heart, from Latin ventriculus (in reference to the heart, ventriculus cordis), literally

"**<u>little belly</u>**," diminutive of venter (genitive ventris) "belly" (see ventral).

The Amduat, Book of Gates, Underworld of Osiris... They are all telling you something, so is modern science. Keep in mind, the same way Hebrew & Arabic come from Mdu Ntr, Modern Science comes from Kemet as well. The Real Christ is your Heart! Which in medicine is viewed electrically PQRST!!! The Wave!!! The Heart stays in the Anointed body!!! It is the messenger of the soul, judged to be Shu-Like!

QRST (Breakdown by letters) - Back of the Head, Apis (Final), Front of the Head, Flag (Most High, Most Important), Shin, 3 Flags (Destroy, Consume), Tau, Nilometer, 19 (Cross, Covenant, Seal)!!!

OK this isn't all random stuff... I just needed you to have all this info first! Look at how your Heart is described Electrically! PQRST!!! That is almost identical to... wait... I didn't tell you???

QRST is the origin of the word Christ, it doesn't come from Christos or Messiah in Hebrew! The Origin of Christ is QRST, sometimes spelled KRST, means buried or the buried one. Yes even Christ comes from Kemet, the Djous! You can just call us the Djous or Djouish people!

The craziest part is the added P, P comes from a Pey/

Fey which represents the Mouth, go back to the IB book!!! Please read &/or reread the IB book, in Kemet they describe the Heart with a mouth, the Heart Speaks.

The Heart is QRST.
The Mouth of the Heart is PQRST.

Look at this from that 12th Dynasty... I told you that may the timeline...

You see it yourself!!! This is all too much even for me! Are you not entertained!!!???

It   would   probably   help   if   yo

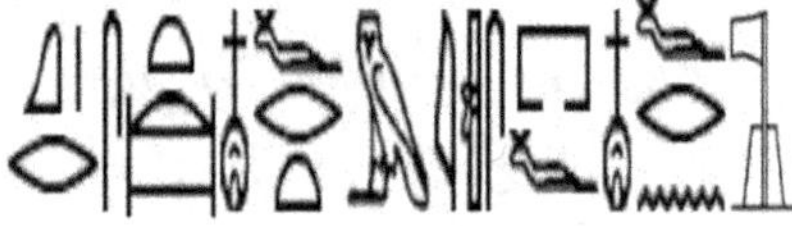

• **12th Dynasty**, coffin of Nakhtankh, *British Museum, Egyptian Antiquities 35285:*

*[...] **qrst** nfrt m jz.f nfr n ḫrt-nṯr [...]*

[...] a good **burial** in his wonderful tomb of the necropolis [...]

u knew what was what huh?

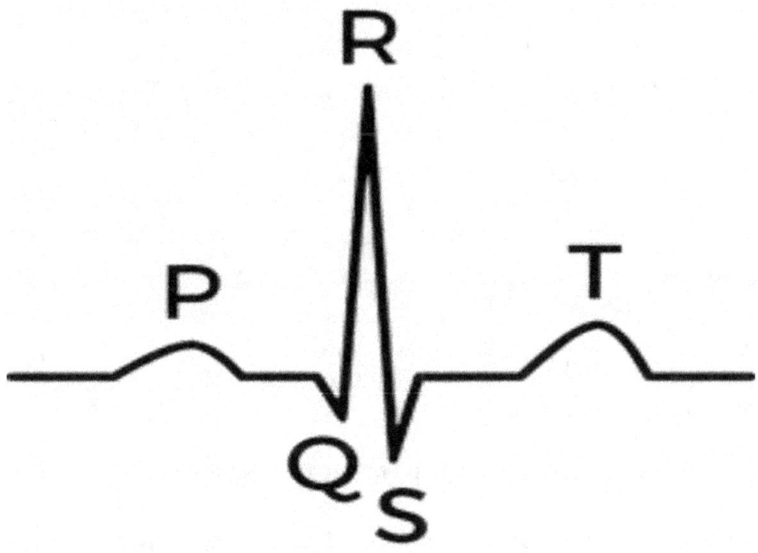

qrst

Entry   Discussion   Citations

Egyptian [edit]

Etymology [edit]

From *qrs* ("to bury") + *-t*.

Pronunciation [edit]

- (*modern Egyptological*) IPA(key): /kɛrɛsɛt/
  - Conventional anglicization: *qereset*

Noun [edit]

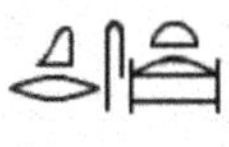

t

1. burial   [quotations ▼]

Mind you what lead me here was studying as a Royal Arch Mason, I was looking for the Holy Royal Arch and it lead me to the Aortic Arch! That lead me to find the Was Scepter as the Aorta....

It also lead me to find the papers buried deep in the annals of Academia that say, your lifespan may be dependent on Melanocytes in the Heart! Yep, the Perfect Black, Osiris once again.

Eu - Good, Well, Perfect

Melanin - Melanos, Black, Brown, Dusky

Even modern Science says that the Heart is the Throne of EuMelanin aka Wusir aka Ausar aka Osiris!

Remember what the Book of Wusir aka the Quran says about the Bible. Wuzir is a figure who is mentioned in the Quran, **Surah at-Tawbah, verse 9:30**, which states that he was "revered by the Jews as the son of God". The Jews say, "Wuzir is the son of Allah," while the Christians say, "The Messiah is the son of Allah." Such are their baseless assertions, only parroting the words of earlier disbelievers. May Allah condemn them! How can they be deluded 'from the truth'?

Now the Question is who exactly do the Jews say is God? Wuzir's father?

ORIGINAL SIN

What exactly is the original sin? The original sin was to become like the Gods. A play on multiple levels, it references the Greeks, becoming like the Gods of Kemet, but also the social science and biochemical science of humans. Humans are the only animals on earth that have the ability to self refer and build tools to extend our fractality. **Fractals** are the geometry of **self reference**. Time, space, light, sound and movement are all in your mind, Heaven & Hell are there too... You can't fully understand the power of the Observer Effect &/or Meditation, definitely not prayer until you get that. Self referral. Think about this the Original Sin is to become like the Gods. Education is to become Godlike, the ability to know Good from Evil. I mean it's that simple, but guess what? Everyone is debating that today! Is gay cool, PDFilia cool? Is it ok to reap the reward from the sweat off the next man brow? Can I tempt the next man into intoxication and then make deals with him... get him to say things... do things...? Can I create poverty and the jail the impoverished for trying to escape poverty? I mean if they don't try to escape poverty legally...forget the fact they are in poverty by illegal means Bwahahahaha... Hypothetically of course... We can drink, just don't get drunk lmao...

Do you know there is a single letter for Sin. The Bible is   soooooo   coded.

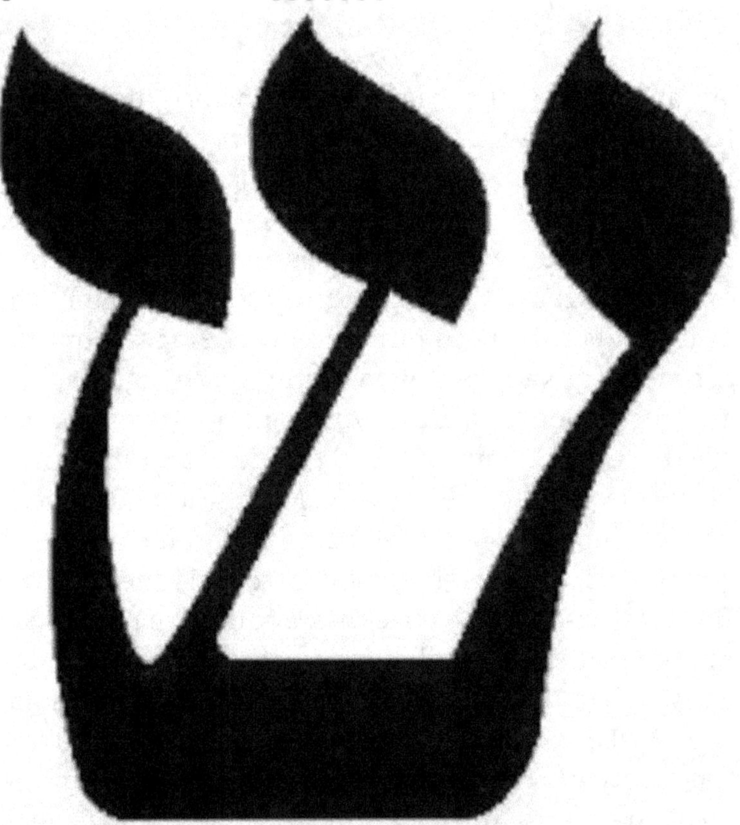

The letter Shin is also the Sin, it makes a S sound and also a Sh sound! It is made after the Neteru sign.

Hebrew letters have inner and outer meanings on top of their numerical values.

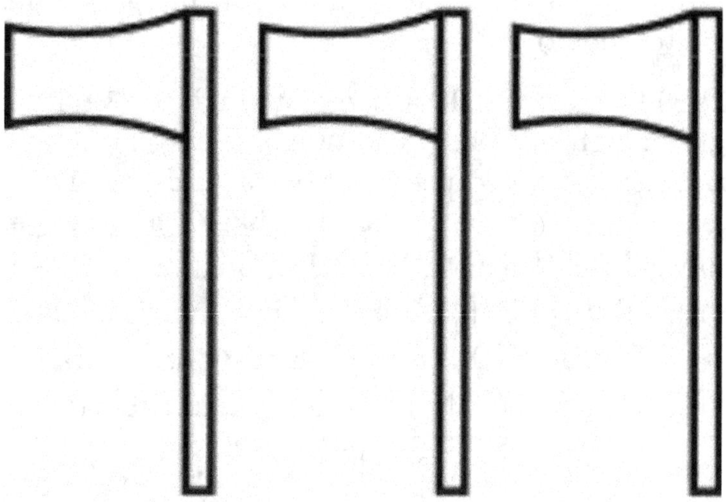

Sin is just like the Gods... Bwahahahahaha... That's nasty work! The funniest part is without Logic and Reasoning you can't get even the low hanging fruit (pun intended)!

The 3 Flags, some still call axes (smdh) is the Kemetic sign for Neteru - Gods. The W looking sign is Sin or Shin, it is tricky because it has two sounds, one like a fire or air and one **like a snake**. HAVING BEEN FORMED FROM ROCK (Dirt is crushed rock) ADAM AND "EVE" REPRESENT THE MENTALLY DEAD ROUGH STONES!!! THERE FORE AS THE DEAD THE NAGGAR OR SNAKE HAD TO TELL THEM HOW TO BECOME GODS!!!

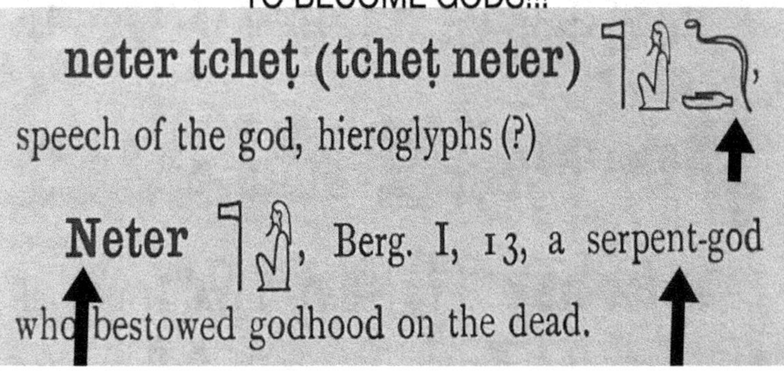

neter tcheṭ (tcheṭ neter) speech of the god, hieroglyphs (?)

Neter , Berg. I, 13, a serpent-god who bestowed godhood on the dead.

Lets walk through the Garden ourselves, now that we all have a taste for Mountain = DJew.

*Genesis the Garden of Egypt, I mean Eden. Eden עֵדֶן [Genesis 2] derives from עֵד "Witness", said to mean Pleasure, Delight, Judge etc... I will say this, there is one spot in the world where a eternal judge lives, that offers pleasure, temptation etc... The Mind, and that is what the Garden is about, the Snake is the Spine and Brain. The **3rd ventricle** actually makes a shooshing sound, especially if you have high blood pressure.

Genesis

And the two were naked, both Adam and his wife, and were not ashamed. Now the serpent was the most crafty of all the brutes on the earth, which the Lord God made, and the serpent said to the woman, Wherefore has God said, Eat not of every tree of the garden?

*CRAFT - SYMBOLIZES THE "CRAFT" OF MASONRY AND INTELLIGENCE!!! THE SAME DESCRIPTION OF **JESUS** AND HIS FATHER, NAGGARS! ISN'T JUST A CO-INCIDENCE THAT **YAHOSHUA** IS CALLED A NAGGAR AND HUNG ON A TREE? I MEAN.... ONLY THE MEN ON EARTH TO RECEIVE THOSE HONORS ARE **YASHUA** AND AMERICAN BLACKMEN.

but of the fruit of the tree which is in the midst of the garden, God said, Ye shall not eat of it, neither shall ye touch it, lest ye die.

*"EVE" WAS CONFUSED, SHE DIDNT UNDERSTAND DEATH WAS SYMBOLIC AND THE TREE WAS INITIATION! SNAKES SYMBOLIZE DEATH, REBIRTH

OR INITIATION. INITIATION IS SIMPLY A WORD FOR INTERNAL EDUCATION & GRADUATION.

**And the serpent said to the woman,
Ye shall not surely die.**

For God knew that in whatever day ye should eat of it your eyes would be opened, and ye would be as Gods, **<u>knowing good and evil</u>**.

*ATOM & "EVENING" GET THE SAME CHOICE THAT SOLOMON WAS GIVEN, PHYSICAL MATERIAL WEALTH (IMMORTALITY) OR KNOWLEDGE AKA LIGHT.

And the woman saw that the tree was good for food, and that it was pleasant to the eyes to look upon and beautiful to contemplate, and having taken of its fruit she ate, and she gave to her husband also with her, and they ate.

*LIGHT IN THE EYES FEED THE SNAKE, HE HUNGERS FOR KNOWLEDGE!!! HE BASICALLY GOT HER TO FEED HIS APPETITE FOR KNOWLEDGE OR CRAFTINESS…

And the eyes of both were opened, and they <u>perceived</u> that they were naked, and they sewed fig leaves together, and made themselves <u>aprons</u> to go round them.

And the Lord God said to the serpent, Because thou hast done this, thou art cursed above all **cattle** and all the brutes of the earth, on thy breast and belly thou shalt go, and thou shalt eat earth all the days of thy life.

*THIS IS NOT A PUNISHMENT, AS MUCH AS A SELF FULFILLING PROPHECY. WHEN YOUR CHILDREN ARE GROWN THEY HAVE TO LEAVE HOME AND TAKE CARE OF THEMSELVES. THE BREAST AND BELLY, IS HUNGER AND INSTINCT, CRAFTINESS. THE MOST HIGHLIGHTED, EATING DIRT ASPECT REFERS TO NUTRITION. WE HAVE TO EAT PROBIOTICS AND MINERALS EVERYDAY. MINERALS ARE LITERALLY, THE DUST OF THE GROUND OR EARTH.

And to the woman he said, I will greatly multiply thy pains and thy groanings; in pain thou shalt bring forth children, and thy submission shall be to thy husband, and he shall rule over thee.

THIS ISNT A CURSE ITS A GIFT, EVE CAN NOT HAVE BABIES AND DOES NOT EVEN HAVE NAME YET!!! EVEN IS A PIECE OF ROUGH CLAY... SHE HAS TO BE PERFECTED, WHICH IS WHAT SHE WAS DOING BY LEARNING GOOD FROM EVIL. EVE DOES NOT HAVE A BELLY BUTTON, NOR DOES ADAM. THIS WAS MORE EDUCATION, BEING GODLIKE ISN'T ALL SWEET, ITS WORK! LOL...

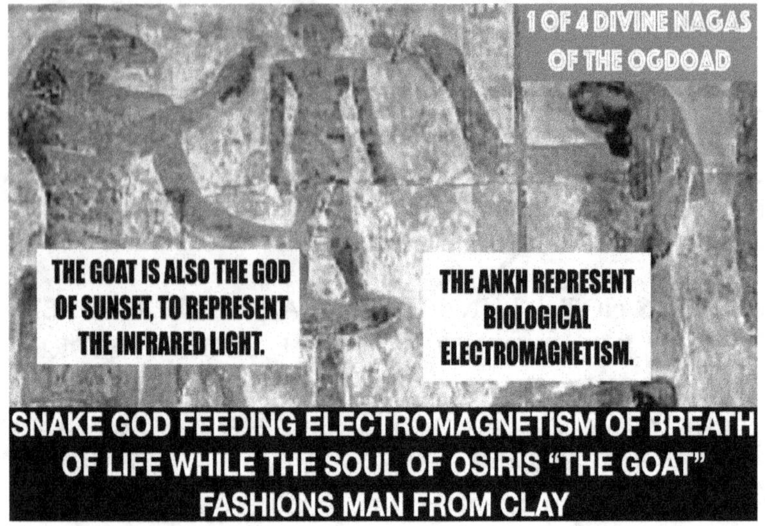

And to Adam he said, Because thou hast hearkened to the voice of thy wife, and eaten of the tree concerning which I charged thee of it only not to eat—of that thou hast eaten, cursed the ground in thy labours, in pain shalt thou eat of it all the days of thy life.

AGAIN NOT A CURSE GOD WAS SIMPLY EXPLAINING TO ADAM THE LIFE OF A GOD. A GOD MUST WORK FOR HIMSELF, FEED HIS FAMILY AND PROTECT THEM... THOSE WERE ALL THINGS "THE GARDEN" TOOK CARE OF!

And Adam called the name of his wife Life, because she was the mother of all living. And the Lord God made for Adam and his wife **garments of skin, and clothed them**.

HERE "THE WOMAN" GETS A NAME AND A CAREER PATH AS A MOM! SHE IS **NAMED AFTER ISIS**! CHAVA (HAWWA) MEANS **TO EXIST**, TO BE ALIVE, TO CREATE LIFE. ISIS FROM THE ROOT ISS MEANING **TO BE TO EXIST TO LIVE**…

THE SAME "ROOT" WE USE TO GET CHIRAM MEAN MUCH LIFE OR EXALTED! THINK ABOUT THIS NEXT TIME YOU HERE L'CHAIM THE CLASSIC TOAST TO LIFE… WAIT WHO DRINKING…LOL THEY WERE ALIVE, SO THEY HAD SKIN BUT THEY WERE NAKED, THEY ALSO NEEDED TO HIDE FROM THE LIGHT BECAUSE OF THIS NAKEDNESS. GOD MAKES THEM AS GODS WITH PIGMENT SO THEY CAN INTERACT WITH THE LIGHT ON THEIR OWN. THIS KNOWLEDGE/LIGHT REQUIRES THE PIGMENT OR SOLOMONS MOSAIC FLOOR… I HAVE HEARD PLENTY OF EXPLANATIONS, LIKE THESE SKINS WERE COATS FOR WARMTH… HOW SWAYE? WHY AT THE EQUATOR WOULD ANYONE NEED COATS? TO ROAM BARREN DESERT LANDS? YES, THIS WOULD IMPLY THAT ADAM & EVE WERE…. ______. CHECK YOUR RACISM!

Just for you the reader…
The Original Sin is Thought, Djehuti, Wisdom. A Sinner is one who knows good from evil, do you see how you have been super tricked? Funny how Djehuti was converted into Thought/Thoth huh?

CHRIST CONSCIOUSNESS

Christ Consciousness is to make you mentally dead. First Christ means buried, burial or one who is buried. That is dead. Secondly, you do not achieve spiritual growth via sex! You can receive spiritual growth via abstinence, by saving yourself, mentally, physically or even withholding ejaculation.

The Satanist had a good thing going, they had celebrities and everything. I mean just like a conspiracy theory movie... Jinn Carey has been on major TV stations promoting sexual brown chakra science. He even added in a splash of PDFilia, he included the kids by saying it's the origin of Santa Clause?!!... Santa is supposed to slide down the chimney and deliver gifts, get it... I won't even go further in what Jinn was describing! These Demons promote this as Christ Consciousness LMAO... How did people allow this to fool them? I will tell you, it's actually simple. The people that turned away from

God allow Checks and Balances, to be their Checks & Balances, get it?

Balance - early 13c., "scales, apparatus for weighing by comparison of mass," from Old French balance "balance, scales for weighing" (12c.), also in figurative sense; from Medieval Latin bilancia, from Late Latin bilanx, from Latin (libra) bilanx "(scale) having two pans," possibly from Latin bis "twice" (from PIE root *dwo- "two") + lanx "dish, plate, scale of a balance," which is of uncertain origin.

The accounting sense "arithmetical difference between the two sides of an account" is from 1580s; the meaning "sum necessary to balance the two sides of an account" is from 1620s. The meaning "what remains or is left over" is by 1788, originally in commercial slang. The sense of "physical equipoise" is from 1660s; that of "general harmony between parts" is from 1732.

Many figurative uses are from the Middle English image of the scales in the hands of personified Justice, Fortune, Fate, etc.; thus in (the) balance "at risk, in jeopardy or danger" (c. 1300). Balance of power in the geopolitical sense "distribution of forces among nations so that one may not dominate another" is from 1701. Balance of trade "difference between the value of exports from a country and the value of imports into it" is from 1660s.

QRST was judged on a Cross, how do I know, how should you know? He rose. The Cross is a reference to the Scale (Judgement), rising is a reference to Shu as well as the empty tomb in the mountain/cave. Keep in mind Christ is also **the Corner Stone Laid in this Mountain**! This hints again to the mountain being ManMade. The tribe of Shu aka of the DJews! To be truly Christlike, is to teach, uplift and care for others. This translates to being Quantumly Entangled with your community and your people. The school system teaches you against that from the moment you enter it. Put school and then money above friends and family. This philosophy fuels the Fibroid business and the Human Trafficking Abortion business!

The Holy Temple is your Body, Churches, Synagogues & Mosques are for harvesting light via Sympathetic Resonance. These edifices are great at creating and sustaining Magnetic Fields. These are beautiful things, they are very powerful, cult is the root word of culture. This is natural for people to come together and build these fields. This is a Hive Mind, great for accomplishing anything! This is what the tower of Babel verses were about, building a edifice that could harness and project thought…

This New Age Christ Consciousness is Slavery to your desires, instincts and hunger. It's the world where Checks and Balances have become Checks and Balances. This is why we Spend Time, Paying

Attention, Balancing our Interest, so we avoid having our Checks & Balances, becoming our Checks & Balances. This is why many popular personalities are currently trying to Save Face. It's better to save our breath, than to save face. We get a infinitely better ROI investing our time in study, prayer, meditation and self referral.

ANOTHER 12

Qrst means refers to the buried one, the perfect black that lives in our Hearts. The name Sah refers to the Father of the Gods (Osiris), as those who pass the weighing of the Heart Ceremony can become Stars. They are still dead in the Western World. In the West Sah would just mean a dead body that has been 'annointed' and prepared.

Man now I have to bring in the Moabites aka Moors...

Moor - "to fasten (a ship) in a particular location by or as by cables, anchors, etc.," late 15c., probably related to Old English mærels "mooring rope," via unrecorded *mærian "to moor," or possibly borrowed from Middle Low German moren or Middle Dutch maren "to moor," from West Germanic *mairojan. Related: Moored, mooring. French amarrer is from Dutch.

"tract of open, untilled, more or less elevated ground, often overrun with heath," c. 1200, from Old English mor "morass, swamp," from Proto-Germanic *mora- (source also of Old Saxon, Middle Dutch, Dutch meer "swamp," Old High German muor "swamp," also "sea," German Moor "moor," Old Norse mörr "moorland," marr "sea"), perhaps related to mere (n.1), or from root *mer- "to die," hence "**dead land**."

The basic sense in place names is 'marsh', a kind of low-lying wetland possibly regarded as less fertile than mersc 'marsh.' The development of the senses 'dry heathland, barren upland' is not fully accounted for but may be due to the idea of infertility. [Cambridge Dictionary of English Place-Names]
Hence moor-fowl "grouse" (c. 1500); moor-hen (mid-14c.); moor-cock (c. 1200 as a surname).

"North African, Berber, one of the race dwelling in Barbary," late 14c., from Old French More, from Medieval Latin Morus, from Latin Maurus "inhabitant of Mauretania" (Roman northwest Africa, a region now corresponding to northern Algeria and Morocco), from Greek Mauros, perhaps a native name, or else cognate with mauros "**black**" (but this adjective appears in late Greek and may as well be from the people's name).

Also applied to the Arabic conquerors of Spain. Being a dark people in relation to Europeans, their name in the Middle Ages was a synonym for "**Negro**;" later

(16c.-17c.), being the name of the nearest Muslims to Western Europe, it was used indiscriminately of Muslims (Persians, Arabs, etc.) but especially those in India. Cognate with Dutch Moor, German Mohr, Danish Maurer, Spanish Moro, Italian Moro. Related: Mooress.

Black - Old English blæc "absolutely dark, absorbing all light, of **the color of soot** or **coal**," reconstructed to be from Proto-Germanic *blakaz "burned" (source also of Old Norse blakkr "dark," Old High German blah "black," Swedish bläck "ink," Dutch blaken "to burn"), from PIE *bhleg- "to burn, gleam, **shine**, flash" (source also of Greek phlegein "to burn, scorch," Latin flagrare "to blaze, **glow**, burn"), from root *bhel- (1) "to shine, flash, burn." The usual Old English word for "black" was sweart (see swart).

The same root produced Middle English blake "pale," from Old English blac "**bright**, shining, glittering, pale;" the connecting notions being, perhaps, "fire" (bright) and "burned" (dark), or perhaps "absence of color." According to OED, in Middle English "it is often doubtful whether blac, blak, blake, means 'black, dark,' or 'pale, colourless, wan, livid' "; and the surname Blake can mean either "one of pale complexion" or "one of dark complexion."
Black was used of dark-skinned people in Old English. Of coffee with nothing added, attested by 1796. The meaning "**fierce, terrible, wicked**" is from

late 14c. The figurative senses often come from the notion of "without light," moral or spiritual. Latin niger had many of the same figurative senses ("gloomy; unlucky; bad, wicked, malicious"). The metaphoric use of the Greek word, melas, however, tended to reflect the notion of "shrouded in darkness, overcast." In English it has been the color of sin and sorrow at least since c. 1300; the sense of "with dark purposes, malignant" emerged 1580s (in black art "necromancy;" it is also the sense in black magic).

Black drop (1823) was a liquid preparation of opium, used medicinally. Black-fly (c. 1600) was a name given to various insects, especially an annoying pest of the northern American woods. Black Prince as a nickname of the eldest son of Edward III is attested by 1560s; the exact signification is uncertain. Black flag, flown (especially by pirates) as a signal of no mercy, is from 1590s. Black dog "melancholy" is attested from 1826.

Black belt is from 1870 in reference to district extending across the U.S. South with heaviest African population (also sometimes in reference to the fertility of the soil); it is attested from 1913 in the judo sense, worn by one who has attained a certain high degree of proficiency. Black power is from 1966, associated with Stokely Carmichael. Black English "English as spoken by African-Americans," is by 1969. The Black Panther (1965) movement was an outgrowth of Student Nonviolent Co-ordinating

Committee. Black studies is attested from 1968.

c. 1200, intransitive, "become black;" early 14c., transitive, "make black, darken, put a black color on;" from black (adj.). Especially "clean and polish (boots, shoes, etc.) by blacking and brushing them" (1550s). Related: Blacked; blacking.

Old English blæc "the color black," also "ink," from noun use of black (adj.). It is attested from late 14c. as "**dark spot in the pupil of the eye**." The meaning "**dark-skinned person, African**" is from 1620s (perhaps late 13c., and **blackamoor** is from 1540s). The meaning "**black clothing**" (especially when worn in **mourning**) is from c. 1400.

To be in black-and-white, meaning in writing or in print, is from 1650s (white-and-black is from 1590s); the notion is of black characters on white paper. In the visual arts, "with no colors but black and white," it is by 1870 of sketches, 1883 of photographs. To be in the black (1922) is from the accounting practice of recording credits and balances in black ink.

For years it has been a common practice to use red ink instead of black in showing a loss or deficit on corporate books, but not until the heavy losses of 1921 did the contrast in colors come to have a widely understood meaning. [Saturday Evening Post, July 22, 1922]

The word for death comes from Mdu Ntr, the crazy

part is they don't have a concept of death. Pronounced the same but spelled different is called Homophone.

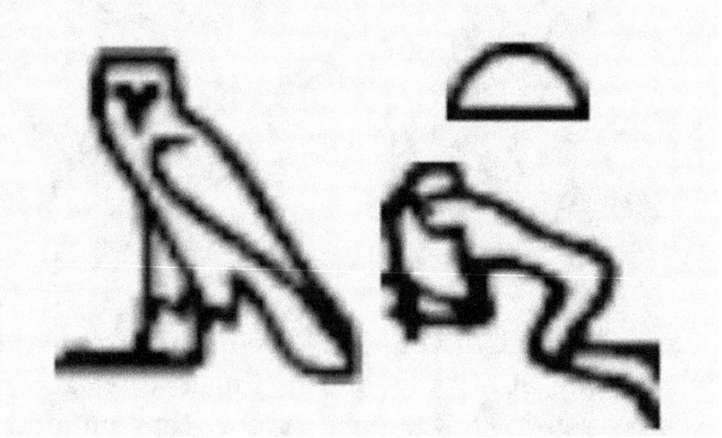

Mut (Ancient Egyptian: mwt; also transliterated as Maut and Mout) was a mother goddess worshipped in ancient Egypt. Her name means mother in the ancient Egyptian language. Mut had many different aspects and attributes that changed and evolved greatly over the thousands of years of ancient Egyptian culture. Think Ammit, Ammit (Ancient Egyptian: m-mwt; ꜣmt mwtw) means "devourer of the dead" ("Devoureress of the Dead") or "Swallower of the Dead". The truth is there was a variety of ways to describe death in the Kemetic sense, just not in a western sense.

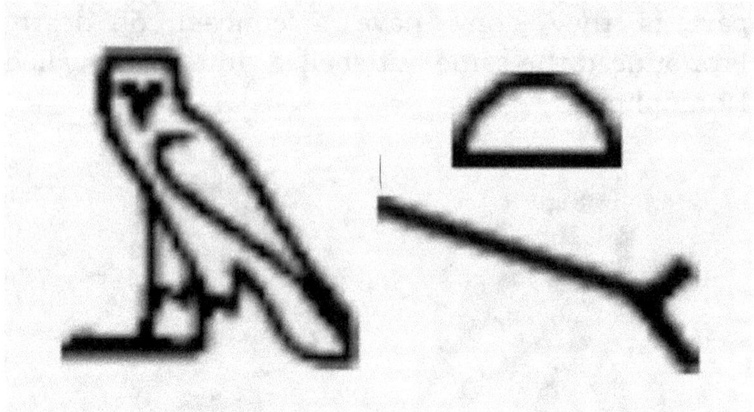

There are some of you that have been laughing this whole time, at least every time I mention death in a western sense. They know that is another entendre… In Kemet falsely called Ancient Egypt, the West was the land of the Dead. The were so far ahead of their time! The Western Culture is the Culture of the Mentally & Spiritually Dead!!! Did they predict this or speak it into existence? I would say predicted since they built the Pyramids to resurrect the Living Dead and Lost Children!

Yeah I am not a Mdu Ntr expert, please go double down and research these mashed up glyphs of mine. The information though, Golden. There really is no concept for the western idea of Dead, a person doesn't really stop living unless they get devoured by Ammit (for flunking the Scales Test). This is why you have to learn to BE IN THIS WESTERN WORLD BUT NOT OF IT!!! This is the world of Golems, 85%

of this world is just Golems. They are mentally and spiritually dead.

Goy - "a gentile, a non-Jew" (plural goyim), 1835, from Hebrew goy "people, nation;" in Mishnaic and Modern Hebrew, also "gentile" (compare gentile). The fem. form of the Hebrew word entered French as gouge "a wench" (15c.).

Golem - "artificial man, automaton," 1897, from Hebrew golem [Psalm cxxxix.16] "shapeless mass, embryo," from galam "he wrapped up, folded."

Your getting real jewels now, God blew his breath in the first Man to create a living soul. After that, Man began making man. Just because your 'alive' does not mean you are a Living Soul. You have the free will to become and act as a Living Soul or be a Westerner. Pay attention as we further uncover your true identity...

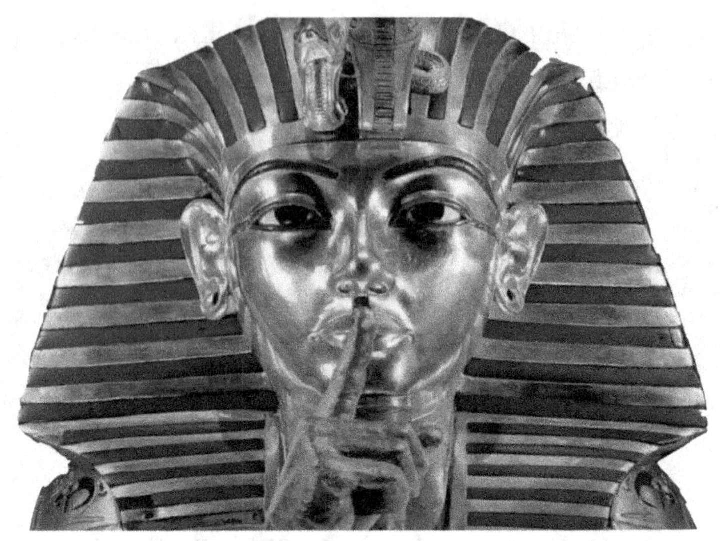

It's our secrets... we the Djews! Ssshhh!

Joseph (/ˈdʒoʊzəf, -səf/; Hebrew: יוֹסֵף, romanized: Yōsēp̄, lit. 'He shall add') is an important Hebrew figure in the Bible's Book of Genesis. He was the first of the two sons of Jacob and Rachel (Jacob's twelfth named child and eleventh son). He is the founder of the Tribe of Joseph among the Israelites. His story functions as an explanation for Israel's residence in Egypt. He is the favourite son of the patriarch Jacob, and his envious brothers sell him into slavery in Biblical Egypt, where he eventually ends up incarcerated. After correctly interpreting the dreams of Pharaoh, however, he rises to second-in-command in Egypt and saves Egypt during a famine. Jacob's family travels to Egypt to escape the famine, and it is through him that they are given leave to settle in the Land of Goshen (the eastern part of the Nile Delta).

The Bible offers two explanations of the name Yosēf: first, it is compared to the triliteral אָסַף (ʾ-s-p), meaning "to gather, remove, take away": "And she conceived, and bore a son; and said, God hath taken away my reproach" (Genesis 30:23); Yosēf is then identified with the similar root יסף (y-s-p), meaning "to add": "And she called his name Joseph; and said, The LORD shall add to me another son." (Genesis 30:24).

Now here is the twist... From the 12th Dynasty again!

The Story of Sinuhe (also referred to as Sanehat or Sanhath) is a work of ancient Egyptian literature. It was likely composed in the beginning of the Twelfth Dynasty after the death of Amenemhat I (also referred to as Senwosret I). The tale describes an Egyptian man who flees his kingdom, and lives as a foreigner before returning to Egypt shortly before his death. It explores universal themes such as divine providence and mercy. The oldest known copy of the text dates to the reign of Amenemhat III, around 1800 BCE. The work was so popular within Egypt that newer copies have been found ranging up to 750 years after the original.

Comparisons have been drawn between the biblical

narrative of Joseph and the Story of Sinuhe. In what is seen as divine providence, Sinuhe the Egyptian flees to Syro-Canaan and becomes a member of the ruling elite, acquires a wife and family, before being reunited with his Egyptian family. Similarly, the Syro-Canaanite Joseph is taken to Egypt where he becomes part of the ruling elite, acquires a wife and family, before being reunited with his Syro-Canaanite family. Then there is the Hebrew prophet Jonah's frustrated flight from the orbit of God's power likened to Sinuhe's similar flight from the King. The battle between David and Goliath is compared to Sinuhe's fight with a mighty challenger, whom he slays with a single blow, and the parable of the Prodigal Son is likened to Sinuhe's return home.

The truth will start becoming clearer and clearer, there is no Egypt/Isreal, only one group of North Africans, Kemetyu. The signal is being sent far and wide, peace and love time is upon us!
We must arrange prayer times! The WaveGuide already has well worn grooves too. We need to get right into the 3-5 times a day habit.

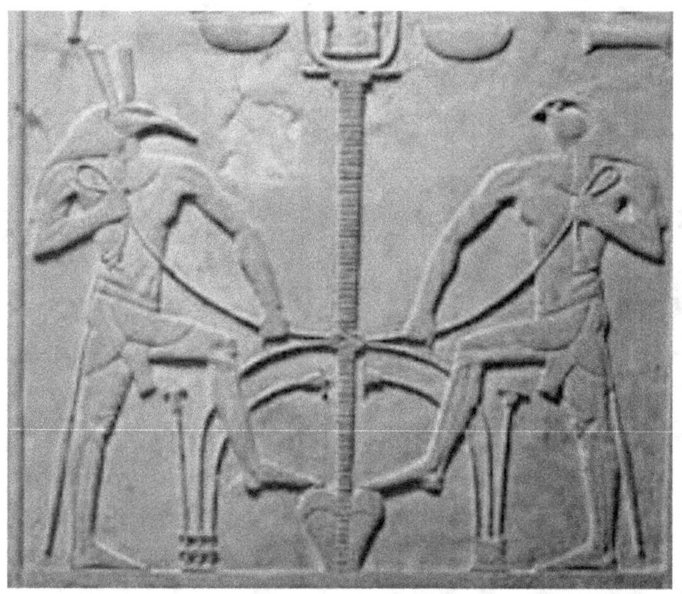

Smai Tawy tied the upper and lower was bigger than politics! It was the Dirt and the Soul, Spirit and Flesh. There is the old issue of the Kaaba, the focus of Islamic prayer. It is wrong, well partially. The direction works because their prayers are powerful and heard. The Kaaba though, it is shirk. Periodt. The reason behind it is simple, the Great Pyramid. Arabic comes from Mdu Ntr, the Ka & Ba are the soul and spirit. That simple. The word Black in Arabic is Aswan, Aswan is a city in Egypt! The word Salah means prayer (to tie one to ALLAH from its root).

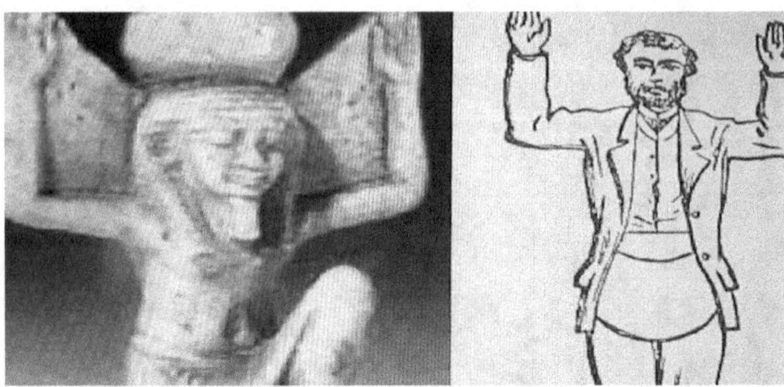

This is no coincidence that the tradition that has the closest definition to Spooky Action at a Distance, has the best prayer system. There are some that even call it contact prayer because your head contacts the Earth (Geb) or because you directly contact Allah (Shu).

In Kemet you also have dua, praise. The Hieroglyph for Dua shows arms raised up, you know who is the God that raises.... A major use of the seated-adoration hieroglyph would be as part of the Libationer-Priest (hieroglyph). Although the main man-seated, adoration hieroglyph is not used in the Rosetta Stone, the Libation-priest is used throughout (beginning at the early lines of the first half of the Decree of Memphis (Ptolemy V), the named Nubayrah Stele). One use on the Rosetta Stone 2nd half of the Libationer-priest is the plural of the priests. The last part of the Decree of Memphis, Ptolemy V-(Rosetta Stone), is to honor Pharaoh Ptolemy by enacting ten items. In the next-to-last line, line R-13, one enactment is:

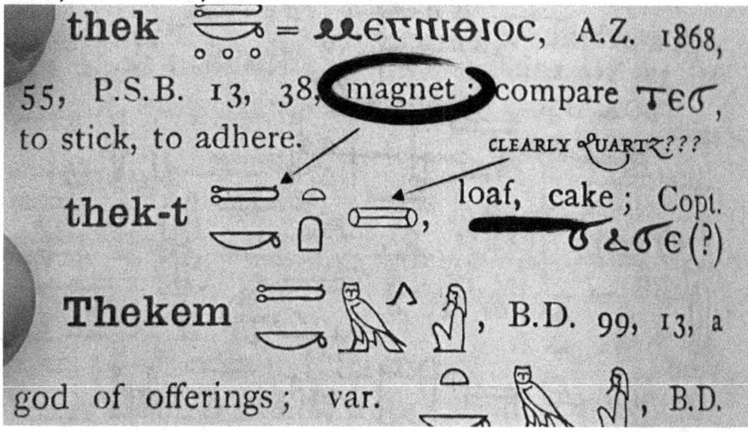

"The priests (Libationer hieroglyphs), of the temples in temple every by its name, shall be called "priest of the god appearing (epiphanous), lord of benefits," (Greek: eucharistos), in addition to the ranks of priests of them (in addition to their other priestly titles). Let write them it upon documents theirs, ..."

This brings us to the Eucharistos, the tradition of Eating the Flesh and Drinking the Blood of Yehoshua. The Arabs sold the mummies for Medicinal Cannibalsim, the religious thing wasn't enough. Yehoshua got hung and he was probably eaten, like many many Black Men, many Christs, in fact all the QRSTs they could find were eaten!!! Do not make any mistake about the Westerners. The bread is supposed to   be   ElectroMagnetism,   not   Flesh.

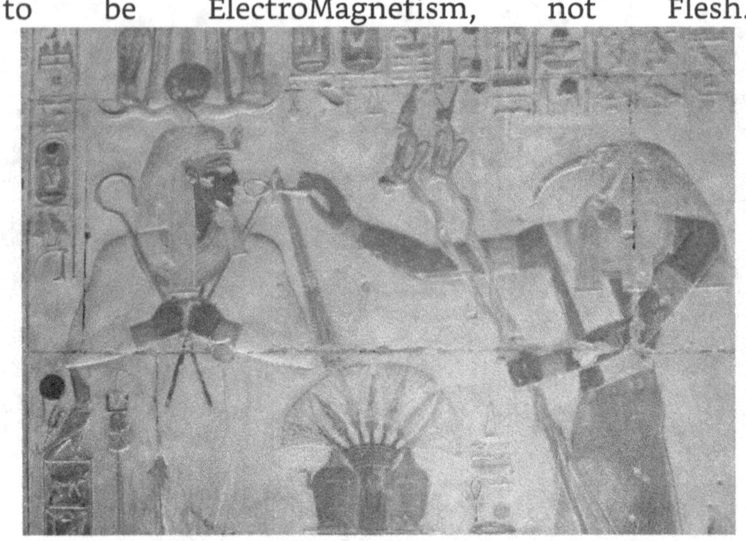

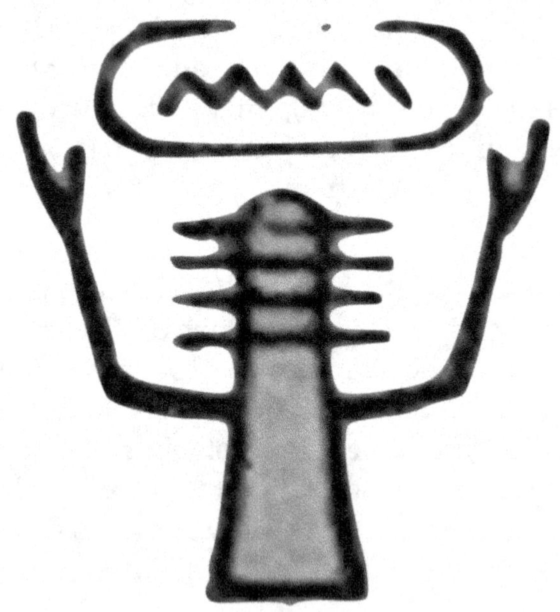

The signal is being transmitted, is your spine healthy? Is your mind drug free?

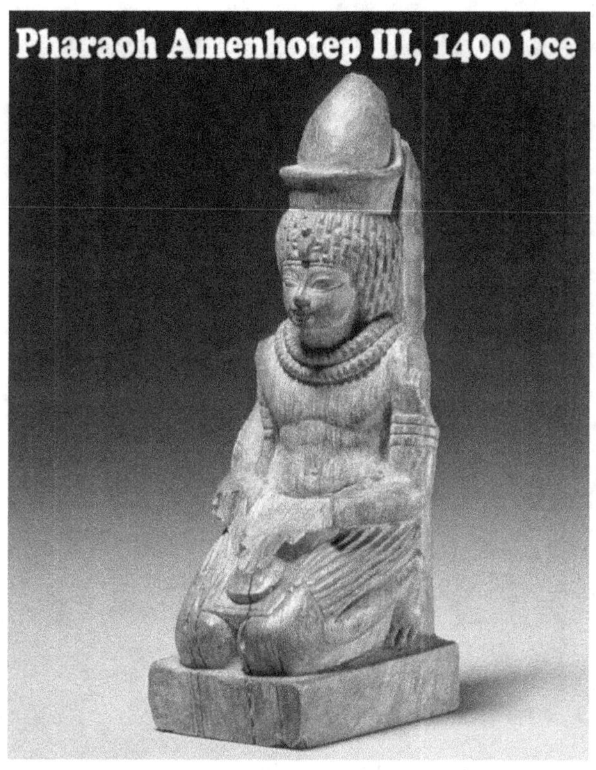

Don't feel any kind of way by praying 3 or 5 times a day. The Arabs are in debt to us, they stole our I.P. and ate our ancestors. We owe them nothing. ʾĀmīn (Arabic: آمِين) is the Arabic form of Amen. In Islam, it is used with the same meaning as in Judaism and

Christianity; when concluding a prayer, especially after a supplication (du'a) or reciting the first surah Al Fatiha of the Qur'an, as in prayer (salat), and as an assent to the prayers of others.

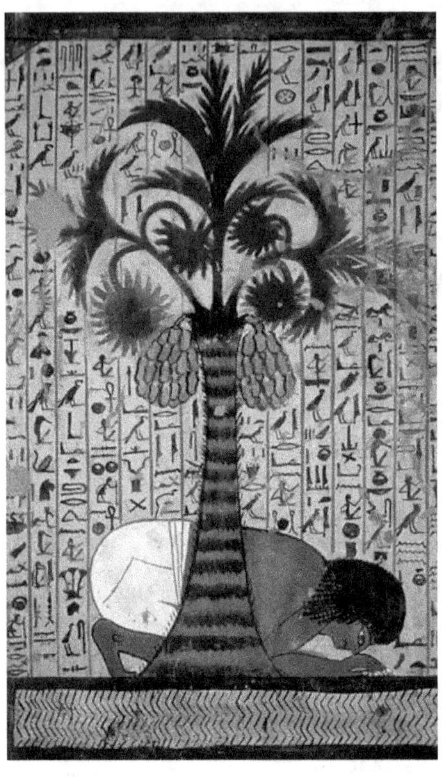

- Fajr: Before dawn - Begins at dawn, may be performed up to sunrise after Fajr nafl prayer

- ZDuhr: At noon - From when the sun has passed the zenith, may be performed up to the time of Asr.

- Asr: In the late afternoon - From when the shadow cast by an object is once or twice its length, may be performed up to the time of Maghrib.

- Maghrib: At sunset - Begins at sunset, may be performed up to the end of dusk.

- Isha: At night - Begins with the night, may be delayed up to dawn although disliked

Yeah then there is that, the midday prayer is actually called Ausar!!! The 'second afternoon' prayer right before 3pm. Notice 3 two 6s and a 12... There is a 5pm prayer but I think it should more accurately be a 9!!! Therefore our prescribed prayer times will be as follows:

- 6am Horus (Ra-Herukhuti/Ra-Horakhty)
- 12pm Shu - the EnQi Prayer (back of this book).
- 3pm Asr
- 6pm Set/Amenti
- 9pm Nun/Isis (bedtime)

Feel free to create your own prayers, please pray for me too. Say the prayers of whatever your religion is, borrow some. You can also say mine all 5 times a day. At the minimum though you should say it once a day at Nun time (12pm). Nun is the cosmic waters that the universe sprang to life from, the blackness of the night sky. This is why we don't call our midday prayer Nun, that is for Shu. Bedtime is when you have better access to Nun. Yes.... I told you its kind covered up but, there is a Joshua who's dad is Nun in the Bible look it up... Nun means Fish... The reason Jesus is often depicted as a fish, the pope's headdress etc... Nun (just kidding that's pure coincidence, it's also a co-inky dink that the cloth needs to be joined at 90 degree angles too).

You need to begin broadcasting purposely! Pray privately or with those in prayer only. If you are at work, school or in public just read/recite your prayer slightly. When in private you need to pray out loud though...! This is will tie you back in tune with all your Ancestors globally. Ask yourself, why did the Indigenous American Chiefs wear Feathers? Shu! Bird like Eagles, Falcons or Quetzals... were all worshiped because of their association with Shu. God of the Air and God of Flight.

Hymn to Osiris Short form...

"Homage to thee, O Osiris, the lord of eternity, the king of the gods, thou who hast many names, whose forms of coming into being are holy, whose attributes are hidden in the temples, whose Double is most august (or venerated). Thou art the Chief of Tettu (or Busiris), the Great One who dwelleth 2.

in Sekhem (Letopolis), the lord to whom praises are offered in the nome of Athi, the Chief of the divine food in Annu (On, or Heliopolis), and the lord who is commemorated in the {Hall (or City) of two-fold Right and Truth. Thou art the Hidden Soul, the lord of Qereret (Elephantine), the holy one in the city of the White Wall (Memphis), the Soul of Ra, and thou art of his own body. Offerings and oblations are made to thy satisfaction in 3. Sutenhenen (Herakleopolis), praise in abundance is bestowed upon thee in Nart, and they Soul hath been exalted as lord of the Great House in Khemennu (Hermopolis). Thou art he who is greatly feared in Shas-hetep, the lord of eternity, the Chief of Abtu (Abydos), thy seat extendeth into the land of holiness (Underworld), and thy name is firmly established in the mouth of mankind. 4. Thou art the substance of {which were made the two lands (i.e., Egypt), thou art Tem, the divine food of the doubles, thou art the chief of the company of the gods, thou art the operative and beneficent Spirit among the spirits, thou drawest thy waters from the abyss of heaven, thou bringeth along the north wind at eventide and air for thy nostrils to the satisfaction of thy heart. 5. Thy heart germinateth, thou producest the light for divine food, the height of heaven and the starry gods obey thee, thou openest the great pylons {of heaven, and thou art he unto whom praises are sung in the southern heaven, and to whom adorations are performed in the northern heaven. The stars which never set 6. are under the seat of thy face, and the stars which never rest are thy habitations; and unto thee offerings are made according to the decree of the god Seb.

Hymn to Osiris long version

"Homage to thee, Osiris, Lord of eternity, King of the Gods, whose names are manifold, whose forms are holy, thou being of hidden form in the temples, whose Ka is holy. Thou art the governor of Tattu (Busiris), and also the mighty one in Sekhem (Letopolis). Thou art the Lord to whom praises are ascribed in the nome of Ati, thou art the Prince of divine food in Anu. Thou art the Lord who is commemorated in Maati, the Hidden Soul, the Lord of Qerrt (Elephantine), the Ruler supreme in White Wall (Memphis). Thou art the Soul of Ra, his own body, and hast thy place of rest in Henensu (Herakleopolis). Thou art the beneficent one, and art praised in Nart. Thou makest thy soul to be raised up. Thou art the Lord of the Great House in Khemenu (Hermopolis). Thou art the mighty one of victories in Shas-hetep, the Lord of eternity, the Governor of Abydos. The path of his throne is in Ta-tcheser (a part of Abydos). Thy name is established in the mouths of men. Thou art the substance of Two Lands (Egypt). Thou art Tem, the feeder of Kau (Doubles), the Governor of the Companies of the gods. Thou art the beneficent Spirit among the spirits. The god of the

Celestial Ocean (Nu) draweth from thee his waters. Thou sendest forth the north wind at eventide, and breath from thy nostrils to the satisfaction of thy heart. Thy heart reneweth its youth, thou producest the.... The stars in the celestial heights are obedient unto thee, and the great doors of the sky open themselves before thee.

Thou art he to whom praises are ascribed in the southern heaven, and thanks are given for thee in the northern heaven. The imperishable stars are under thy supervision, and the stars which never set are thy thrones. Offerings appear before thee at the decree of Keb. The Companies of the Gods praise thee, and the gods of the Tuat (Other World) smell the earth in paying homage to thee. The uttermost parts of the earth bow before thee, and the limits of the skies entreat thee with supplications when they see thee. The holy ones are overcome before thee, and all Egypt offereth thanksgiving unto thee when it meeteth Thy Majesty. Thou art a shining Spirit-Body, the governor of Spirit-Bodies; permanent is thy rank, established is thy rule. Thou art the well-doing Sekhem (Power) of the Company of the Gods, gracious is thy face, and beloved by him that seeth it. Thy fear is set in all the lands by reason of thy perfect love, and they cry out to thy name making it the first of names, and all people make offerings to thee. Thou art the lord who art commemorated in heaven and upon earth. Many are the cries which are made to thee at the Uak festival, and with one heart and voice Egypt raiseth cries of joy to thee.

"Thou art the Great Chief, the first among thy brethren, the Prince of the Company of the Gods, the stablisher of Right and Truth throughout the World, the Son who was set on the great throne of his father Keb. Thou art the beloved of thy mother Nut, the mighty one of valour, who overthrew the Sebau-fiend. Thou didst stand up and smite thine enemy, and set thy fear in thine adversary. Thou dost bring the boundaries of the mountains. Thy heart is fixed, thy legs are set firm. Thou art the heir of Keb and of the sovereignty of the Two Lands (Egypt). He (Keb) hath seen his splendours, he hath decreed for him the guidance of the world by thy hand as long as times endure. Thou hast made this earth with thy hand, and the waters, and the winds, and the vegetation, and all the cattle, and all the feathered fowl, and all the fish, and all the creeping things, and all the wild animals therof. The desert is the lawful possession of the son of Nut. The Two Lands (Egypt) are content to crown thee upon the throne of thy father, like Ra.

"Thou rollest up into the horizon, thou hast set light over the darkness, thou sendest forth air from thy plumes, and thou floodest the Two Lands like the Disk at daybreak. Thy crown penetrateth the height of heaven, thou art the companion of the stars, and the guide of every god. Thou art beneficent in decree and speech, the favoured one of the Great Company of the Gods, and the beloved of the Little Company of the Gods.

His sister [Isis] hath protected him, and hath repulsed the fiends, and turned aside calamities (of evil). She uttered the spell with the magical power of her mouth. Her tongue was perfect, and it never halted at a word. Beneficent in command and word was Isis, the woman of magical spells, the advocate of her brother. She sought him untiringly, she wandered round and round about this earth in sorrow, and she alighted not without finding him. She made light with her feathers, she created air with her wings, and she uttered the death wail for her brother. She raised up the inactive members of whose heart was still, she drew from him his essence, she made an heir, she reared the child in loneliness, and the place where he was not known, and he grew in strength and stature, and his hand was mighty in the House of Keb. The Company of the Gods rejoiced, rejoiced, at the coming of Horus, the son of Osiris, whose heart was firm, the triumphant, the son of Isis, the heir of Osiris."

When I was a practicing Muslim back in my late 20s, I was so proud to have this memorized!

Make the intention of praying then raise hands to ears and say:
Allaahu Akbar (Allah is the greatest!)
Subhaanaka Allaahumma wabi hamdika wa

tabaarakasmuka wa ta'aala jadduka wa laa ilaaha ghayruka.
Glory be to You, O Allah, and all praises are due unto You, and blessed is Your name and high is Your majesty and none is worthy of worship but You.
  A'oodhu billaahi minash-Shaytaanir-rajeem
I seek Allah's protection from Satan the accursed.

Bismillaahhir-Rahmaanir-Raheem
In the name of Allah, the Most Compassionalte and the Most Merciful.

Alhamdul lillaahi rabbil 'aalameen; Ar-rahmaanir-raheem; Maaliki yawmiddeen; Iyyaaka na'budu wa iyyaaka nasta'een; Ihdinas-siraatal mustaqeem; Siraatalladheena an'amta 'alayhim; ghayril maghdubi 'alayhim; waladdaal-leen. Ameen
Praise is only for Allah, Lord of the Universe; The most Compassionate, the Most Merciful; The Master of the Day of Judgement; You alone we worship and to You alone we pray for help; Show us the straight path, the path of those whom You have blessed, who have not deserved Your wrath, nor gone astray.

Qul huwallaahu 'ahad, Allaahus-Samad. Lam yalid walam yoolad. Walam yakullahu kufuwan ahad.
Say: He is Allah, the Only One. Allah helps and does not need help. He did not produce a child, and He was not born of anyone. There is no one equal to Him.

Subhaana Rabbi-yal Azeem: "Glory to my Lord the Exalted".

Sami'a Allaahu liman hamidah: "Allah listens to him who praises Him":

Rabbanaa lakal hamdu: Oh our Lord, all praise is to You. Subhaana Rabbiyal A'alaa: "Oh Allah, glory be to You, the Most High."

Athahiyyaatu lillaahi was-salawaatu wattayyibatu. Assalamu 'alaika ayyuhan-nabiyu warahmatullaahi wabarka'tuhu. Assalamu 'alaina wa'alaa 'ibaadillaahis saa'liheen. Ash'had'u alla ilaha illallahu wa ash'hadu anna Muhammadan abd'uhu ea rasooluh.

All compliments, all physical prayer and all worship are for Allah. Peace be upon you, O 'Prophet, and Allah's mercy and blessings be on you. Peace be on us and on all righteous slaves of Allah. I bear witness that no one is worthy of worship except Allah and I bear witness that Muhammad is His slave and Messenger.

Allaahumma salle 'alaa Muhammadin wa'alaa' aale Muhammadin kama sallaiyta 'alaa Ibraheema wa 'aAlaa Aale Ibraheema. Innaka Hameedum Majeed. Allaahumma baarik 'alaa Muhammadin wa 'alaa aale Muhammadin kama baarakta 'ala Ibraheema wa 'alaa Aale Ibraheema. Innaka Hameedum Majeed.

Oh Allah, send grace and honour on Muhammad and on the family and true followers of Muhammad just as you sent Grace and Honour on Ibrahim and on the family and true followers of Ibrahim. Surely, you are praiseworthy, the Great. Oh Allah, send your blessings on Muhammad and the true followers of Muhammad, just as you sent blessings on Ibrahim and his true followers. Surely, you are Most Praiseworthy, the Exalted.

Assalamu 'alai'kum warah'matullaah: Peace and mercy of Allah be on you.

DR.ENQI

Raw Herbal Compounds
PRODUCT GUIDE

Detox Kit:

Kemeluminescence -
NRF2, YEAST, FUNGUS, FAT SUPPORT;
Bladderwrack, Yarrow, Cascara Sagrada, Moss, Happy Tree, Madagascar, Periwinkle, Mayapple, Pacific Yew, Cloves, Amla, Coriander, Black Walnut, Kelp, White Pine Bark, Horny Goat Weed, Milk Thistle, Tribulus, Bitter Melon, Chaste Berry, African Pygeum, Cinnamon, Gynesylvestre, Hemp, Pau D Arco, African Bird Pepper, Cinchona Bark, Chinese Senega Root, Biden Pilosa, Houttuynia, Licorice, Skullcap, Scute Root, Ginseng, Rehmania, Er Bu Shir Tao, Bugleweed

Swadj Momatomix -
Marrow & Electromagnetism Support / Rich in Hydrogen, Phosphorus, Aromatic Amino Acid Phosphorus, Nettles, Wild Lettuce, Hydrogen, Plant Enzyme, &Alkaloid+ MATRIX

Antiviral Kit -

Antiviral
Antifungal
Antibacterial
mtDNA Protector
The most comprehensive organic antiviral kit ever assembled to fight viral infection and improve recovery

Antivirals -
Exogenous & Endogenous Pathogen Support
Cilantro, Celery, Chaparral, Olive Leaf, Oregano Leaf, Black Walnut, Lysine, Tyrosine, Thyme, Cleavers, Hyssop, Bladderwrack, Ginger

Antiviral Nutrient -
Pathogen Suppression Support
Manganese, Rosemary, Hydrangea, Bilberry, Rhizome Rei

Antiviral Oil -
Immunglobulin & Antibody Support
Oregano, Peppermint, Tea Tree, Cinnamon, Hyssop, Thyme, Clove, Ginger

Calcium -
Muscle & Bone Support
Blood Pressure, Insulin Control, Nerve Function, Muscle Contraction
Kelp, Calcium, Sesame, Cloves

Chromium & Vanadium -

Glucose Tolerance Factor & Eyesight Support
Fat Loss , Insulin Metabolism , Hydration , Muscle
Integrity , Energy
Chromium, Fenugreek, Vanadium, Bitter Melon,
Gymnema Sylvestre

Copper -
Pigment System Support
Cardiovascular Key, Heart Beat Nutrient, White
Blood Cell Reg
Copper, Cilantro, Cloves, Milk Thistle

Iron -
Heme & Magnetism Support
Electron Circulation, Digestive System,
Thermogenesis, Brain Power
Iron, Yellow Dock, Stinging Nettles, Chaparral

Magnesium -
Energy & Light Metabolism Support
Muscle Function, Energy, Builds ; Proteins/ Enzymes/
Hormones , DNA Repair
Blue Vervain, Burdock, Parsley, Magnesium

Muscle Drip -
Children/Adults Multivitamin & Bone Tendon
Compound
Blood Oxygen, Breakdown Lactic Acid, Builds Blood
Cells Faster, Cleans Lymphatic System
Elderberries, Cherries, Sea Moss, Stinging Nettles,
Horsetail, Lily of the Valley, Bladderwrack, Bromide,

Melatonin, Phosphorus, Boron, Calcium, Strontium

Muscle Plants -
Children + Adults Multivitamin & Muscle/Joint Compound
Gout, Autography, Enhanced Healing, Arthritis, Remove Stones
Elderberries, Cherries, Bugleweed, Hombre Grande, Blue Vervain, Chaparral, Ginseng, Rhodiola, Boswellia, Eluethero, Melatonin, Phosphorus, Magnesium

Selenium -
Immune Plasma Support
Thyroid Health, Cancer Suppression, Mental Health, Tumor Suppression
Selenium, Burdock, Bladderwrack, Sarsaparilla

Swadj Momatomix -
Marrow & Electromagnetism Support / Rich in Hydrogen, Phosphorus, Aromatic Amino Acid
Phosphorus, Nettles, Wild Lettuce, Hydrogen, Plant Enzyme, &Alkaloid+ MATRIX

Zinc -
Skin & Enzyme Support
Anabolic Boost, Immune System Nutrient, Stem Cell Health, Gene Support
Rosemary, Chlorella, Sage, Zinc

Watermelanin -
Nootropic, Dopamine, Muscle Recovery, Nourish

Your Pineal Gland, DMT Support
Raw Organic Non-GMO Black Watermelon Seeds
Lupulin

Anabolic Hormone Help -
Anabolic Hormones, AMPK & Circadian Support
Jiaogulan, Wild Lettuce, Tribulus, Longjack, Maca &
Pollen Blend

Histonic -
Histone Sirtuin Support
Grape Skin, Resveratrol, Tyrosine Analogue, Japanese
Knotweed

Ocean Steak -
Vegan B12, Carbon, Nucleoside, Protein, Nucleotide,
Omega 3 & Eye Support
Phytoplankton, Duckweed, Chlorella, Purple Laver,
Chondrus Crispus & C60 Lutein, Zeaxanthin, Ocean
Pigment Matrix

Chrondris Crispus -
Structured Water Mucus Membrane Support
Copper, Cilantro, Cloves, Milk Thistle

NON GMO Moringa -
Whole Body Nutrition Support
Raw Organic Non-GMO Moringa

Purple Phaze -
Anti-Aging Longevity Support
FoTi, Pumpkin Seed, NMN, Bhringaraj, Biotin, Silica,
Tyrosine, Yucca, White Willow Bark, French Lilac,

NAD

Every item on this list, every compound is not only from God but works on the skin from the inside out, what we need now is topical.

Topical = Tropical

Batana is Great but it's expensive and incomplete.

Researchers identify 135 new melanin genes responsible for pigmentation

Date: August 11, 2023

Source: University of Oklahoma

Summary: The skin, hair and eye color of more than eight billion humans is determined by the light-absorbing pigment known as melanin. New research has identified 135 new genes associated with pigmentation. Vitamin D and Vitamin A... I told you nature doesn't wait to be discovered before getting to work! Melanin vs Diabetes as a Ministry & Movement isn't waiting around to save lives... We have saving lives and creating thought leaders for 20 years!!! The thing is science just discovered 135 genes for pigment and melanin, how the F@3$ have the been acting as if.... This is why we rely on Nature, God & our Ancestors.

We are teaching the world, showing the world...

#HealingLooksLikeThis

Most people don't know what the process of Healing actually Looks Like!!!

People judge health by how your skin looks, literally your complexion. Your Complex of Ions!

Complexion - the general aspect or character of something; the natural color, texture, and appearance of a person's skin, especially of the face.

complexion (n.)
mid-14c., complexioun, "temperament, natural disposition of body or mind," from Old French complexion, complession "**combination of humors**," hence "temperament, character, make-up," from Latin complexionem (nominative complexio) "combination" (in Late Latin, "physical constitution"), from complexus "surrounding, encompassing," past participle of complecti "to encircle, embrace," in transferred use, "to hold fast, master, comprehend," from com "with, together" (see com-) + plectere "to weave, braid, twine, entwine," from PIE *plek-to-, suffixed form of root *plek- "to plait."
The Middle English sense is from the old medicine notion of bodily constitution or general nature resulting from blending of the four primary qualities (hot, cold, dry, moist) or humors (blood, phlegm, choler, black choler). The specific meaning

"**<u>color or hue of the skin of the face</u>**" developed by mid-15c. In medieval physiology, the color of the face was believed to be caused by the balance of humors in the body and indicate temperament or health. The word rarely is used in the sense of "state of being complex."
also from mid-14c.

Humor - the quality of being amusing or comic, especially as expressed in literature or speech; a mood or state of mind. **Each of the four chief fluids of the body (blood, phlegm, yellow bile (choler), and black bile (melancholy)) that were thought to determine a person's physical and mental qualities** by the relative proportions in which they were present.

humor (n.)
mid-14c., "**fluid or juice of an animal or plant**," from Old North French humour "liquid, dampness; (medical) humor" (Old French humor, umor; Modern French humeur), from Latin umor "body fluid" (also humor, by false association with **humus "earth"**); related to umere "**be wet**, moist," and to uvescere "become wet" (see humid).
In old medicine, "any of the four body fluids" (blood, phlegm, choler, and melancholy or black bile).

*The human body had four humors—blood, phlegm, yellow bile, and black bile—which, in turn, were associated with particular organs. Blood came from the heart, phlegm from the brain, yellow bile from the liver, and black bile from the spleen. Galen and Avicenna attributed certain elemental qualities to each humor. Blood was hot and moist, like air; phlegm was cold and moist, like water; yellow bile was hot and dry, like fire; and black bile was cold and dry, like earth. In effect, the human body was a microcosm of the larger world. [Robert S. Gottfried, "The Black Death," 1983]

Their relative proportions were thought to determine physical condition and state of mind. This gave humor an extended sense of "mood, temporary state of mind" (recorded from 1520s); the sense of "amusing quality, funniness, jocular turn of mind" is first recorded 1680s, probably via sense of "whim, caprice" as determined by state of mind (1560s), which also produced the verb sense of "indulge (someone's) fancy or disposition." Modern French has them as doublets: humeur "disposition, mood, whim;" humour "humor." "The pronunciation of the initial h is only of recent date, and is sometimes omitted ..." [OED].

For aid in distinguishing the various devices that tend to be grouped under "humor," this guide, from Henry W. Fowler ["Modern English Usage," 1926] may be of use:

HUMOR: motive/aim: discovery; province: human nature; method/means: observation; audience: the sympathetic

WIT: motive/aim: throwing light; province: words & ideas; method/means: surprise; audience: the intelligent

SATIRE: motive/aim: amendment; province: morals & manners; method/means: accentuation; audience: the self-satisfied

SARCASM: motive/aim: inflicting pain; province: faults & foibles; method/means: inversion; audience: victim & bystander

INVECTIVE: motive/aim: discredit; province: misconduct; method/means: direct statement; audience: the public

IRONY: motive/aim: exclusiveness; province: statement of facts; method/means: mystification; audience: an inner circle

CYNICISM: motive/aim: self-justification; province: morals; method/means: exposure of nakedness; audience: the respectable

SARDONIC: motive/aim: self-relief; province: adversity; method/means: pessimism; audience: the self

also from mid-14c.

We alway have to remember the Greeks were educated by the Egyptians, ie...

Eu - Good, Perfect, Complete

Melanin (Melanos) - Black

EuMelanin is the new way to reference Osiris.

The new usage of humor came from state of mind, which came from your health, based in the balance of fluids.

#StayWet

The herbs and bitters are to condition the internal fluids, the BleuMagick conditions the body's waters, we are now going to top it off with #SkinFood, to make sure you can #StayWet.

Please read &/or reread Lymphatic Immunity, Mitochondria Water, HydroChemistry...

You've got to learn everything you can from these books about Water. Then you will be ready to apply these principles and practices, Kitchen Chemistry, Orthorexia & this book espouse! Truth be told, these 3 books are plug and play immediately... but the further study is what refines you. You have to disappear sometime and come back stronger. You don't that by consuming new information in your absence.

The biggest difference between those in the Rat Race, and those who aren't, is Priority of Consuming New Information. Reading.

What does it mean to you that, the other pigments in the skin control Melanin production?

What does it mean to you that, they just discovered 3000 new types of Neurons?

Neurons are either specialized Melanocytes or Melanocytes are specialized Neurons, they have discovered 3,000 new types Naga.... Wake Up!!! Either your whole body is a Brain or a Heart! The Heart has all of these cells, Neurons, Nerves, Melanocytes etc...

What does it mean to you that, they just discovered 135 genes that are associated with Pigment? Is that 135 genes for the Skin? Brain? Heart???

My goal is to make #SkinFood inexpensive enough for you and your family to use twice a day, that way we can #StayWet.

In L'Goat we explain in detail how water builds what it needs, with the right conditions. First thing is well, Water. Second thing obviously is Retinoids, to fertilize the soil. Then of course Sunlight...

You are the Dust of the Ground, Divine Soil, remember that the ground exerts pressure on seeds. You need the proper exercise, to create that mechanical pressure to stimulate growth and regeneration. Mechanical Pressure helps to circulate Magnetism, this is the #BleuMagick of #ElectroMagneticTissue.

If this is your first book of ours that you have read... God Bless Eu, or maybe this isn't your first book but you haven't read PiezoElectroChemistry, please do that...

You are the Fruit of Melanin, your S.elf O.rganizing U.niversal L.ight.

Soul is the Fruit of PhotoVoltaic Pigment.

The Bible has many allusions to the **Sun** and its 12 houses, but they replace the Sun with the Son. The Bible is full of Truth, full of Science, you just have to know what your looking at. Kemetic Science is a mixture of Photochemistry, Photobiology & Acoustics. The key is remembering that Light and Sound only exist in your mind. The electromagnetic spectrum you are used to seeing is deceptive, so I have taken the liberty to provide you with a more straight forward version in this book.

ElectronVolts - an electronvolt (symbol eV, also written electron-volt and electron volt) is the measure of an amount of_**kinetic energy** gained by a single electron accelerating from rest through an electric potential difference of one volt in vacuum, 1 eV equal to the exact value 1.602176634×10−19 J, a unit of energy or work, **the work required to move an electron** through a potential difference of one volt. 1 eV would correspond to an infrared photon of wavelength 1240 nm or frequency 241.8 THz.

4-12 ELECTRON VOLTS = UVC 100-320 NM DEATH WM

3.9 ELECTRON VOLTS = UVB SKIN 290-320 NM

DISEASE JW

3.4 ELECTRON VOLTS = UVA 320-400 NM EYE DISEASE SW

.001 ELECTRON VOLTS = FAR INFRARED 1000000 NM BEYOND THIS POINT IS RADIO WAVES

.4 ELECTRON VOLTS = NEAR FAR INFRARED 3000 NM

.8 ELECTRON VOLTS = MEDIUM INFRARED 1500 NM

1.5 ELECTRON VOLTS = NEAR INFRARED 780 NM

1.7 ELECTRON VOLTS = VISIBLE RED 620-780 NM

2 ELECTRON VOLTS = VISIBLE ORANGE 585-620 NM

2.1 ELECTRON VOLTS = VISIBLE YELLOW 570-585 NM

2.3 ELECTRON VOLTS = VISIBLE GREEN 490-570 NM

2.6 ELECTRON VOLTS = VISIBLE BLUE 440-490 NM

2.9 ELECTRON VOLTS = VISIBLE INDIGO 420-440 NM

3 ELECTRON VOLTS = VISIBLE VIOLET 400-420 NM

We will look at the E.M. Spectrum in terms of Electron Volts, this makes more sense because all of chemistry is based on the movement of electrons. The Sun is the great visible agent of the first cause. This of course means you have to rethink the whole entire ElectroChemistry aka Dr. Sebi vs Dr. EnQi book…

Sound Range: 20 to 20,000 Hz

Voice Range 90 to 255 Hz

Radio Range: 1 hertz up to 3,000 billion hertz. Below Radio is Cellular, Extremely low frequency (ELF) electric and magnetic fields (EMF) occupy the lower part of the electromagnetic spectrum in the frequency range 0-100 kHz. ELF EMF result from electrically charged particles.

Infrared Range 1 Trillion Hertz to … this is where our body heat is…

TECHNOLOGY EQUIPMENT RECAP

HydroGenes - 1! Proton and 1! Electron.

Melanocytes - Photovoltaic Cells

Neurons/Nerves - Electromagnetic Cells

Fascia - Plasma Medium (misonomered Ether)

Brain - CPU, Inductor

Brainstem - Two-way Adapter for CPU into the Motherboard

Pineal Gland - Receiver, Crystal Tuner & Actuator Arm/Head responsible for Phosphorescence, Thermoluminescence, Piezoelectricity, Birefringence & Harmonic Generation (very much like the otoconia in the ears)

Operating System - Deductive Logic or PQ

<u>Heart</u> - Hydraulic Ram, Turbine (from the Greek τύρβη, tyrbē, or Latin turbo, meaning vortex) and Hard Drive.

<u>Melanosomes</u> - Alternators

<u>Mitochondria</u> - Motors

<u>Myelin Sheath</u> - Insulation

<u>Cytoskeleton</u> - Filaments

<u>Phospholipids</u> - Capacitors, Dielectric Material (lipids in general)

<u>Spine</u> - Piezoelectric, Motherboard, Radio Wave Antenna

<u>RBC</u> - Floppy Discs

<u>Lymph Nodes</u> - Filters, Nodes

<u>Tastebuds</u> - Electronic Scanners

<u>Protein</u> - Transformer

<u>Transformers 'Roll Out'</u> - Conformational Change (Macromolecule Shape Shifting)

<u>Antioxidants</u> - Semi-conductors (especially the selenium based...)

<u>Body Cells</u> - Plasma based Crystal disc, fitted with integrated circuits as well as gates and channels (see Human Cell Membrane and/or Computer Chip)

<u>Nerves & Vessels</u> - 'Copper' wires (CoAxial Cables) and Fiber Optics

<u>Pigment, Nerve & Blood Clusters</u> - Input Devices like a Mouse, Keyboard, etc...

<u>DNA</u> - Piezoelectric, Antenna, Data Storing Inductors.

DNA sub entry **<u>Tissues</u>** - Short Living Stories.

DNA sub entry **<u>Genome</u>** - Substrate & Product, a digital Library (HardDrive) of all your Ancestors have ever seen, said, touched, tasted or heard.

DNA sub entry **<u>Chromosome</u>** - Rewritable Unlimited Storage Books (Folders) of the Library, DNA.

DNA sub entry **<u>Histone</u>** - Writing instrument, encoders and **book spines**.

DNA sub entry **<u>non-coding RNA</u>** - Self Organizing Books Shelves

DNA sub entry **<u>Gene</u>** - Chapters (Files) in the Books, source codes.

DNA sub entry **<u>Messenger RNA</u>** - Protein Information, a Sentence.

DNA sub entry **<u>Codon</u>** - Word (Binary Code there are 2 bonds between each 3 nucleotides representing their arrangement), Amino Acid.

DNA sub entry **<u>Nucleotide</u>** - Letter

DNA sub entry **<u>Nucleoside</u>** - Bits of Information

<u>Collagen Based Tissue</u> - Piezoelectric Inductors

<u>Stomach</u> - Chemical Mixer

<u>Lumen</u> - the SI unit of luminous flux = to the amount of light emitted per second..... or hollow structures in vessels and cells... hmmm????

<u>Eyes</u> - Camera Lens/Charge Coupled Device (CCD), Digital to Analogue Converter, Complex Photovoltaic Cells/Photodetector...

<u>Amino Acids</u> - Fuses that can be almost anything!

<u>Nucleic Acid</u> - Actual Intelligence (self powering too).

<u>N-Type Semiconductors</u> - Selenium or Silica doped with Phosphorus (Alkaline-ish)

<u>P-Type Semiconductors</u> - Selenium or Silica doped with Boron (Acid-ish)

<u>PN Junction</u> - <u>Crystal Lattice Structure</u> Material allowing the flowing of electrons in one direction.

<u>Bone and Fascia</u> seem to be a massive N-Type, P-Type, PN Junction Super computer on it's own... especially if we add in the Piezoelectricity & Vitamin D!

<u>Rectifier</u> - N-Type + P-Type + PN Junction in Bone

<u>Melanin</u> - CPU Core, Solar Repeater

<u>Human Cell Membrane and/or Computer Chip</u> - A flat semiconducting (crystal) disc or wafer, with integrated circuits (resistors/conductors) and/or gates & channels. We now have to add the filaments into this Crystal Disc we call a Body Cell or Somatic Cell.

<u>Transistors</u> - a semiconductor device with three connections, capable of amplification in addition to rectification.

The location that a virus goes viral in, is called a **<u>Hotspot</u>**? WTH!

<u>Virus</u> - an infective agent that typically consists of a nucleic acid molecule in a protein coat, is too small to be seen by light microscopy, and is able to multiply only within the living cells of a host.

Wait you see that, it is happening again! Host...

See look there is another definition of **<u>Virus</u>** - a piece of code that is capable of copying itself and typically has a detrimental effect, such as corrupting the system or destroying data.

Wait a damn minute! DNA is a piece of **<u>code</u>**... A viral strand of DNA or RNA that can jump host is fully capable in that context of copying itself, one would even argue, that is it's only 'motion'. The detrimental effects of corrupting the system (physical illness) or destroying data (mental illness), can clearly be seen anthropomorphically.

Alien - Virus

Culture - the arts and other manifestations of human intellectual achievement regarded collectively, the customs, arts, social institutions, and achievements of a particular nation, people, or other social group. The cultivation of bacteria, tissue cells, etc. in an artificial medium containing nutrients, a preparation of cells obtained from a culture. The cultivation of **plants**.

Going Live - become operational.

Live Stream - a live transmission of an event over the internet, transmit or receive live video and audio coverage of (an event) over the internet.

The Web - Arachnoid Mater

Download - copy (data) from one computer system to another, typically over the internet, an act or process of downloading data.

Upload - transfer (data) from one computer to another, typically to one that is larger or remote from the user or functioning as a server, an act or process of downloading data.

Data - facts and statistics collected together for reference or analysis; the quantities, characters, or symbols on which operations are performed by a computer, being stored and transmitted in the form of electrical signals and recorded on magnetic, optical, or mechanical recording media.

Host - an animal or plant on or in which a parasite or commensal organism lives. VS

Host - store (a website or other data) on a server or other computer so that it can be accessed over the internet.

Transmission is the act of transferring something from one spot to another, like a radio or TV broadcast, or a disease going from one person to another.

I am highlighting the unknown and proposing we may have some answers! <u>Infection - an infectious disease.</u>

plural noun: infections "a chest infection"

Vs

Infection - the presence of a virus in, or its introduction into, a computer system. What is a computer system?

Computer System - a computer system is a programmable electronic device that can accept input; store data; and retrieve, process and output information.

<u>Pandemic language = Virology/Biology language.</u>
The question is, why? The next question is what does that have to do with Dr. Sebi or Robert Becker? The obvious....

<u>Computer System</u> - a computer system is a programmable electronic device that can accept input; store data; and retrieve, process and output information.

<u>Computer System</u> - a single information processor but usually a group of processors that have specified and general computations; grouped by hardware ie... liver cells, lung cells, brain cells etc.. What you think?

<u>Exercise</u> - activity requiring physical effort, carried out to sustain or improve health and fitness.
"exercise improves your heart and lung power"

<u>Exercise</u> - computer training or computer based training.

<u>Exigenetics</u> - Term created by Dr. EnQi for Melanin vs Diabetes research, denoting the control that exercise has over gene expression.

<u>Hydration</u> - the process of inducing gelling, ionizing, dissolution & turbulent flow with activation of cytochrome c (via infrared light).

<u>Resonance</u> - the quality in a sound of being deep, full, and reverberating. "the resonance of his voice"

- The ability to evoke or suggest images, memories, and emotions."the concepts lose their emotional resonance"

- The reinforcement or prolongation of sound by reflection from a surface or by the synchronous vibration of a neighboring object.

- The condition in which an electric circuit or device produces the largest possible response to an applied oscillating signal, especially when its inductive and its capacitative reactances are balanced.

- The condition in which an object or system is subjected to an oscillating force having a frequency close to its own natural frequency.

- The occurrence of a simple ratio between the periods of revolution of two bodies about a single primary.

- The state attributed to certain molecules of having a structure that cannot adequately be represented by a single structural formula but is a composite of two or more structures of higher energy.

- • A short-lived subatomic particle that is an excited state of a more stable particle.

Induction - the action or process of inducting someone to a position or organization."the league's induction into the Baseball Hall of Fame"

Induction - a formal introduction to a new job or position.plural noun: inductions
"an induction course"
enlistment into military service.

Induction - The process or action of bringing about or giving rise to something."isolation, starvation, and other forms of stress induction" the process of bringing on childbirth or abortion by artificial means, typically by the use of drugs.

Induction - The inference of a general law from particular instances.

Induction -"the admission that laws of nature cannot be established by induction" the production of facts to prove a general statement.

Induction - a means of proving a theorem by showing that if it is true of any particular case it is true of the next case in a series, and then showing that it is indeed true in one particular case.

Induction - noun: mathematical induction; plural noun: mathematicals inductionthe production of an electric or magnetic state by the proximity (without contact) of an electrified or magnetized body.

Induction - The production of an electric current in a conductor by varying the magnetic field applied to the conductor.

Induction - The stage of the working cycle of an internal combustion engine in which the fuel mixture is drawn into the cylinders.

Is there anyone reading this that would disagree with our body fitting these definitions, the definitions of a computer?

Man this thought experiment just got a lot more interesting didn't it? MIT and the US Military are different types of receipts huh? Is it possible frequency resonance, spreads disease? Human modems? Can Shedding be a broadcast signal?

Wi-Fi is a wireless networking technology that uses radio waves to provide wireless high-speed Internet access. A common misconception is that the term **Wi-Fi** is short for "wireless fidelity," however Wi-Fi is a trademarked phrase that refers to IEEE 802.11x standards.

<u>Viral shedding</u> is a term for when viruses are replicating or reproducing, the virus is being led out of the host cell where it's replicating or reproducing ... Viral shedding is the expulsion and release of virus progeny following successful reproduction during a host cell infection. Once replication has been completed and the host cell is exhausted of all resources in making viral progeny, the viruses may begin to leave the cell by several methods.

<u>Vaccine</u> - a substance used to stimulate immunity to a particular infectious disease or pathogen, typically prepared from an inactivated or weakened form of the causative agent or from its constituents or products.

<u>Vaccine</u> - a program designed to detect computer viruses and inactivate them.

"the rate of use of vaccines for computer viruses is not as high as in the US, Japan, and other countries"

<u>Application</u> - a medicinal substance put on the skin.

<u>Application</u> - a program or piece of software designed and written to fulfill a particular purpose of the user.

In our thought experiment, if a virus is simply the

media for harmful information...

<u>Media</u> - an intermediate layer in the wall of a blood vessel or lymphatic vessel.

<u>Media</u> - the main means of mass communication (broadcasting, publishing, and the internet) regarded collectively.

<u>DOPE</u> - an illicit drug (such as heroin or cocaine) used for its intoxicating or euphoric effects especially : MARIJUANA (dopamine altering)

<u>Dope</u> - a preparation (such as an anabolic steroid, diuretic, or tranquilizer) given to a racehorse to help or hinder its performance

<u>To Dope</u> - In semiconductor production, to dope is the intentional introduction of impurities into an intrinsic semiconductor for the purpose of modulating its electrical, optical and structural properties. The doped material is referred to as an extrinsic semiconductor.

<u>Short Circuit</u> - Cardiac Arrest?

<u>Short Circuit</u> - Multiple Sclerosis (due to loss of insulation)

<u>Overheating</u> - Fever?

<u>Overcurrent</u> - Inflammation

With Infection and Virus included we are onto

something.

<u>Current</u> - belonging to the present time; happening or being used or done now.

<u>Current</u> - <u>a body of water</u> or air <u>moving in a</u> *definite* <u>direction</u>, especially <u>through a surrounding body of water</u> or air in which there is less movement.

<u>Current</u> - a flow of electricity that results from the ordered directional movement of electrically charged particles.

<u>Current</u> - a quantity representing the rate of flow of electric charge, usually measured in amperes.

<u>Current</u> - the general tendency or course of events or opinion.

<u>Leakage Current</u> - the unintended loss of energy, gain of resistance or results of faulty/worn out insulation.

<u>Plasma</u> - Electric Currents or Electric Current Carrier

<u>Electric Current</u> - Magnetic Field (AtomSphere) Carrier

<u>Alternating Magnetic & Electric Waves</u> - Light

<u>NeuroTransmitters</u> - Record of ElectroMagnetic Waves produced by Neurons (ElectroChemical Message)

Hormones - Large simple versions of NeuroTransmitters (ElectroChemical Message)

Malware - External Negative Mental Programming

Food - Informative Electronic Batteries

0) Movement and sound create energy from water for basic cellular function, via the EnQi Cycle which includes Mitochondria Water. This system slowly increases as all other energy systems fail.

1) Phosphocreatine - anaerobic (no respiration required), phosphocreatine donates it "phospho" to ADP to recycle ATP. This makes 10 ATP per second, its a 1 to 1 ratio (1 phosphocreatine creates 1 ATP) and this is the jump start energy.

2) Anaerobic Glycolysis - anaerobic (no respiration required), Glycogen &/or Glucose to Lactate, 5 ATP per second, 1 to 3 ratio (1 Glycogen creates 3 ATP while 1 Glucose creates 2 ATP) and this is bulk of the energy we focus on, 9 - 120 seconds.

3) NAD/Cytochrome 1 - aerobic (requires oxygen), Glycogen &/or Glucose to CO_2/H_2O, 2.5 ATP per second, 1 to 38 ratio (1 Glycogen &/or Glucose creates 38 ATP), 2 minutes up to 2 hours.

4) FAD/Cytochrome 2 - aerobic (requires oxygen), FFA &/or Triglycerides to CO_2/H_2O, 1.5 ATP per second, 1 to 360 ratio (1 Glycogen &/or Glucose creates 360 ATP), 2 minutes up to 2 days.

Food rule of thumb - Resynthesis of ATP of Inverse to Yield, the closer the ratio is to 1:1 the fast it can be recycled.

Muscle rule of thumb - Frequently used muscle is slow twitch, Fast twitch is slowly used (at that's the blueprint).

Electric Power - the **rate** at which work is done or energy is transformed into an electrical circuit. Simply put, it is a measure of how much energy is used in a span of time.

Conductor - a person who directs the performance of an orchestra or choir.

Conductor - a material or device that conducts or transmits heat, electricity, or sound, especially when regarded in terms of its capacity to do this.

Lymphatic System - Watermill

Circulatory System - Generator

Integumentary System - Photovoltaic Diaphragm

Immune System - Antivirus, Malware Scanner, Frequency Filter & Rectifier

Nervous System - Power Transmission and Cellular Communications Lines

<u>Fascia System</u> - HydroElectric Grid, Scaffolding

<u>Respiratory System</u> - Windmill

<u>Windmill</u> - a structure that converts wind power or "air" power into rotational energy or vortex energy, to mill grain. In our case grain is Magnetism!

MAGNETS ARE DEFINED BY GRAINS
MAGNETIC GRAINS ARE DEFINED BY APPLIED
STRESS AND CRYSTAL GEOMETRY
SPM SUPERMAGNETIC
SD SINGLE DOMAIN
PSD PSEUDO DOMAIN
MD MULTIDOMAIN

<u>Reproductive System</u> - Quine (self-replicating programs)

<u>Skeletal System</u> - Piezoelectric Crystal Shaped to produced highly specific frequency under stress, Dynamic Oscillators.

<u>Urinary System</u> - Industrial Wastewater, Return Flow, Surface Runoff, Urban Runoff Agricultural & Animal Husbandry Wastewater

<u>Digestive System</u> - Massive Inductor

<u>Mouth</u> - Industrial Grinder

<u>Endocrine System</u> - Programmer for Human Cell Membrane and/or Crystal Gel Computer Chips

<u>Human Being</u> - Resonator

<u>Vessels</u> - Pipes

<u>Aromatic Ring</u> - Cyclotron (Particle Accelerator)

<u>Glycation</u> - Corrosion

<u>Exegenetics</u> - Holistic Biomechanics; the purposeful science of combining light, water, diet & exercise to effect DNA.

<u>EnQi's 1st Law of Metabolism</u> - The conversion rate of cholesterol should match the activity of Melanin in the skin. These two systems are designed to be and stay coupled. A dark skin person with low sunlight intake and low exercise is going to die from a Metabolic Complication. The only time Animal Flesh is safe to be consumed by a Eumelanin Dominant person is in times of starvation or extremely high activity.

This Law is a Constant and when broken results in disease every time.

<u>EnQi's 2nD Law of Metabolism</u> - The average rate of applied mechanical stress on the bone electrically stimulating bone marrow, determines the rate of bone deterioration and Red Blood Cell production.

<u>EnQi's 3rd Law of Metabolism</u> - The human body metabolizes Transverse Waves and Mechanical Waves into Electricity. Electricity is the main driver of Biochemistry. Exercise is just as potent a driver of Biochemistry as the Sun.

EnQi's 4th Law of Metabolism - Electron movement and bonding is the Nature of Chemistry. PhotoChemistry and PiezoElectroChemistry are the Primary drivers of Biochemistry.

The Ancients discovered this and created Martial Artforms as a way to clean the Bone, Bone Marrow & Brain. Plaque & Sugar are the top drivers of Brain Disease. The things destroying the Heart are secondarily destroying the brain, and they are the breaking of these Universal Laws.

EnQi's 5th Law of Metabolism - Nutrients are actually substrates that must be transformed via biochemistry to be meaningful. This means that providing your body with lots of nutrition without the Water, Light & Exercise don't work alone.

EnQi's 6th Law of Metabolism - The Body maintains the least amount of bone marrow required to handle blood demand. The marrow is very energy demanding, thus attracting and storing fat for energy, eventually becoming fat itself. Fatty bone marrow is called yellow bone marrow. Yellow Bone Marrow can be reconverted to Red Bone Marrow should the body's demands require it, and the body's resources facilitate it. The primary driver is pressure, hormesis training on the Bones. BMR is heavily driven by Bone Marrow, this means Bone Marrow is a driver if insulin and insulin resistance.

<u>EnQi's 7th Law of Metabolism</u> - The system of pigments throughout the body are for metabolism of Light, actual Soulfood. The Adsorption & Absorption of Photons by Water.

Adsorption - increase in the concentration of a dissolved substance at the interface of a condensed and a liquid phase due to the operation of surface forces.

Absorption - a physical or chemical phenomenon or a process in which atoms, molecules or ions enter some bulk phase – liquid or solid material. This is a different process from adsorption, since molecules undergoing absorption are taken up by the volume, not by the surface.

<u>EnQi's 8th Law of Metabolism</u> - in a diabetic state, sugar is simply invisible to the body. Sugar is not being "sensed" because it's not being converted to energy. In this state of starvation the body turns on every pathway it has to produce sugar from everything you have in your body, fats and proteins included.

This is the reason that it seems like no matter what you eat or 'don't eat', your blood sugar goes up. It's very frustrating. The only way to make it stop is converting that substrate (glucose) into it's final product (energy). The reception of the actual energy, tells the body to stop producing substrate, we good. This must start in the legs and back, the largest muscles but most overlooked. The legs are particularly punished by sitting for extended periods of time, 3-6 hours straight, for a total over 3/4 the time your awake! The leg circulation atrophies and destroys the nerves, nerves are neurons that need a lot of nutrients!

*You must cross reference any and all protocols; food, exercise, medication etc... with the Constitution book & Declaration of Independence!

EnQi Prayer
Hail SHU who Created the Heavens & the Earth, Hail Wusir who gave us Pigment.
And there was Electromagnetic Waves, before and beyond our pigment created Light, for which we give thanks.
And there was Mechanical Waves, before and beyond our pigment created Sound, for which we give thanks.
And there is heat, for which we are grateful.
And there is power, for which we are grateful.
Blessed be Tefnuit & Nuit, for giving us a womb made of water.
Blessed be Shu & Geb, who gave us ElectroMagnetism.
Blessed be Djehuti, who gave us wisdom.
Blessed be Atum-Re, who gave us sight.
We give thanks for the Blessings of Shu.

Blessed are we for cellular E.L.F waves, so our cells can talk to each other.

Blessed are we for long radio waves, which oscillate slowly.

Blessed are we for broadcast waves, for which we educate & communicate with via Djed Pillars natural and handmade.

Blessed are we for short waves, linkers of humankind.

Blessed are we for microwaves, that we may sea better.

Blessed are we for infrared, bearers of nourishing heat and Melatonin.

Blessed are we for visible light, tuned to our waters.

Blessed are we for red, sacred to Set.

Blessed are we for orange (dark yellow there was no orange in Kemet), sacred to the Rising Sun.

Blessed are we for Khenet (yellow), hallowed by Re's gaze.

Blessed are we for sWadj (green), the color of our skin, gift from Wusir.

Blessed are we for Khesbedj (lazuli Blue), for its hydrogen line and recycling Vitamin A.

Blessed are we for Irtyu (indigo), which tricks us by looking mefkhat (turquoise) sometime.

Blessed are we for violet, flourishing with energy.

Blessed are we for ultraviolet, which creates Melanin & Vitamin D.

Blessed are we for X rays, sacred to stone, that we

may sea better.

Blessed are we for the gamma, dangerously high vibrations.

We give thanks for the Geniuses Tesla, Mesmer, Swan, Brush, Planck, Einstein, Thomas, Heaviside, Steinmetz, West, Brown (a sister), Easley (a sister), Morgan (Black Edison), Latimer, Sampson, Russell, Turner, Sebi, Becker and others that re-membered the body of Shu-Amun for us.

In light of Light and Sound, in light of Electromagnetic Waves, Mechanical Waves and the Holy Trinity, Amen!

BOOKS

40 DAY FRUIT FAST
TAPWATER IS
HEALTHIER
THAN SODA
WRITTEN BY:
Chase DuQuesnay Dr. EnQi ReaL
AMERICAN HEALER
RESPECT THE HEALER
NOT THE SHOOTER

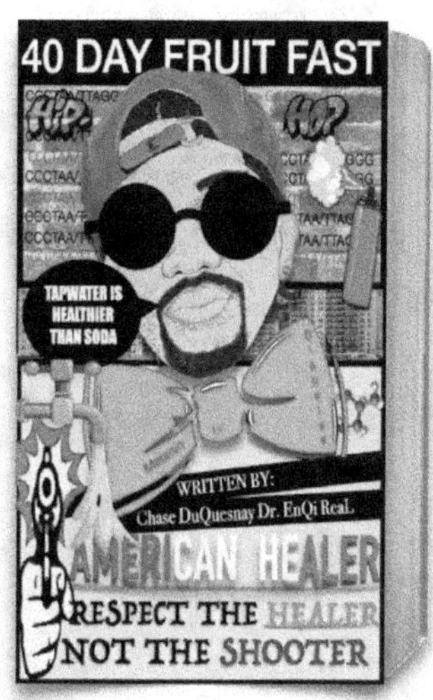

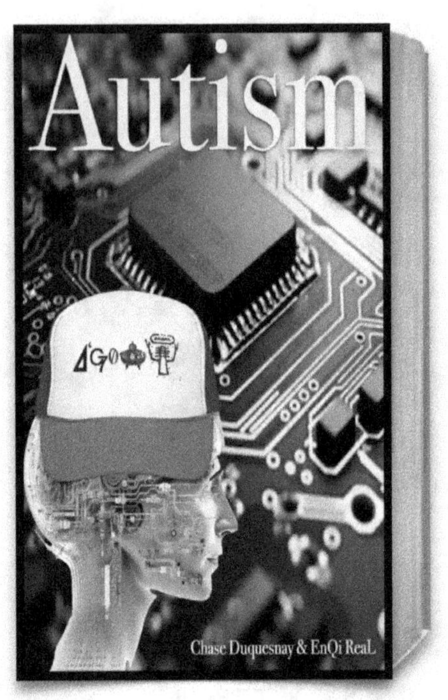

Autism
Chase Duquesnay & EnQi ReaL

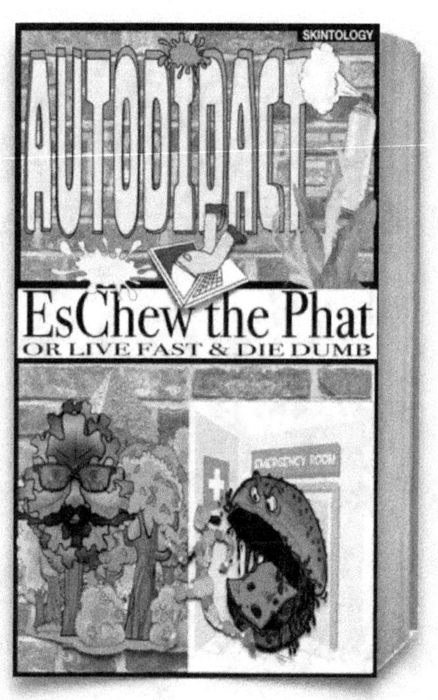
SKINTOLOGY
AUTODIPACT
EsChew the Phat
OR LIVE FAST & DIE DUMB
EMERGENCY ROOM

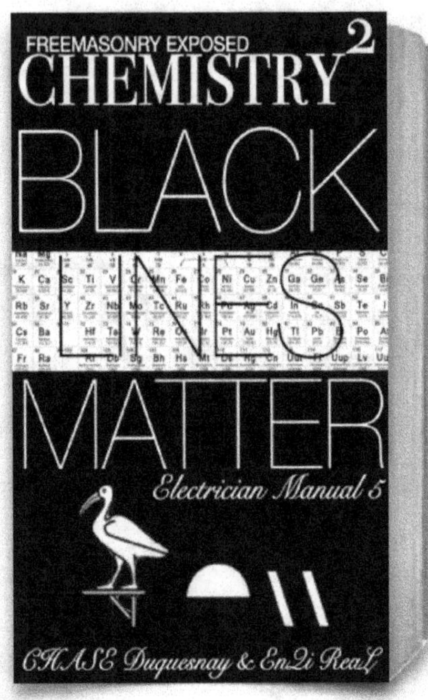

FREEMASONRY EXPOSED
CHEMISTRY 2
BLACK
LINES
MATTER
Electrician Manual 5
CHASE Duquesnay & En2i ReaL

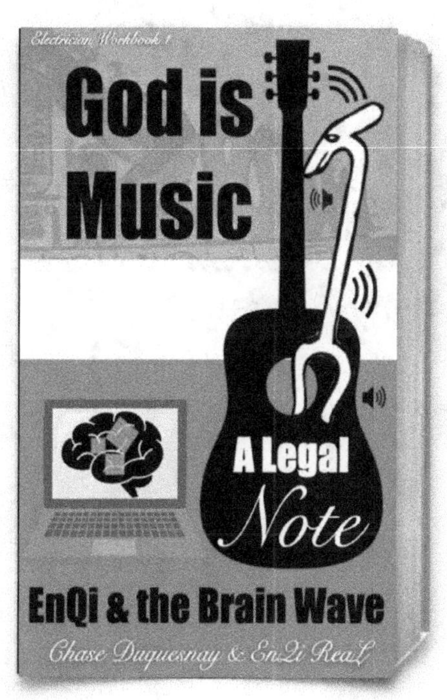

Electrician Workbook 1
God is Music
A Legal
Note
EnQi & the Brain Wave
Chase Duquesnay & En2i ReaL

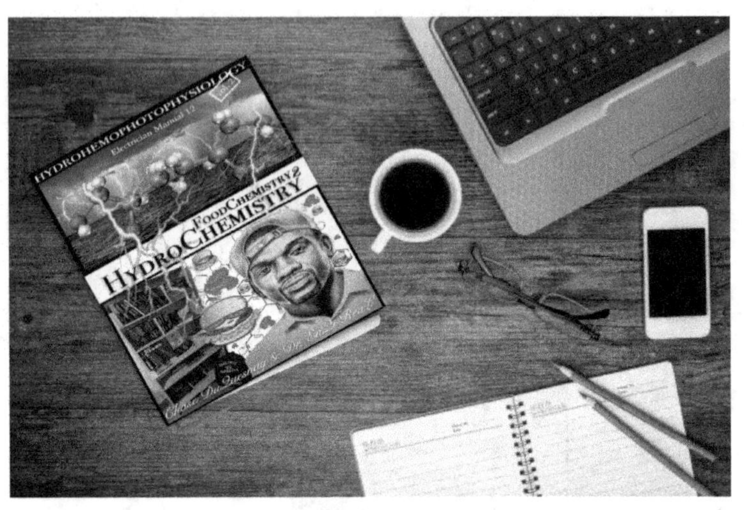

HYDROHEMOPHOTOPHYSIOLOGY
Electrician Manual V2
FoodChemistry2
HydroChemistry

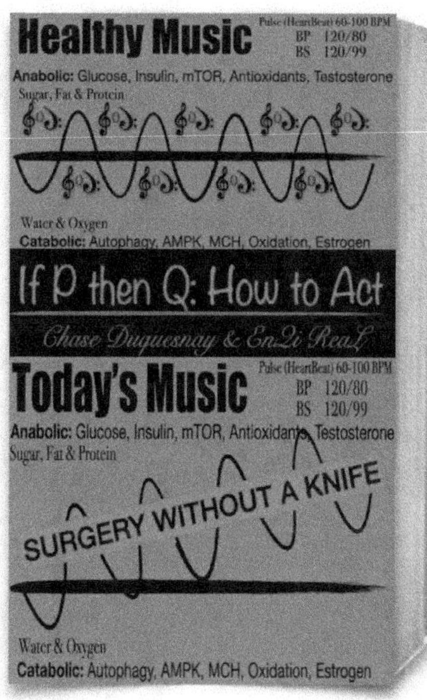
Healthy Music
Pulse (HeartBeat) 60-100 BPM
BP   120/80
BS   120/99
Anabolic: Glucose, Insulin, mTOR, Antioxidants, Testosterone
Sugar, Fat & Protein
Water & Oxygen
Catabolic: Autophagy, AMPK, MCH, Oxidation, Estrogen
If P then Q: How to Act
Chase Duquesnay & En2i ReaL
Today's Music
Pulse (HeartBeat) 60-100 BPM
BP   120/80
BS   120/99
Anabolic: Glucose, Insulin, mTOR, Antioxidants, Testosterone
Sugar, Fat & Protein
SURGERY WITHOUT A KNIFE
Water & Oxygen
Catabolic: Autophagy, AMPK, MCH, Oxidation, Estrogen

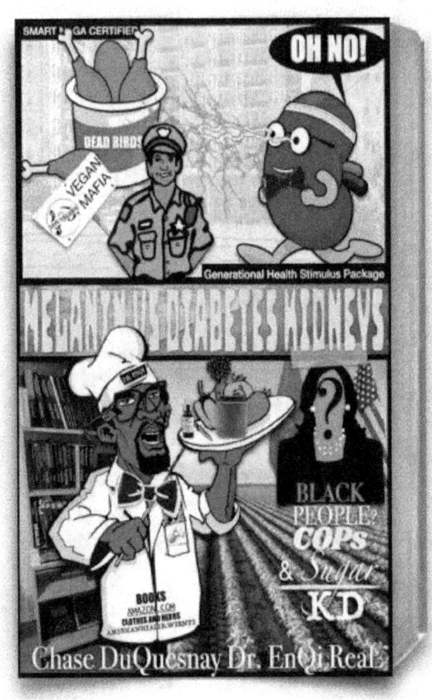

SMART MAGA CERTIFIED
OH NO!
DEAD BIRDS
VEGAN MAFIA
Generational Health Stimulus Package
MELANIN VS DIABETES KIDNEYS
BOOKS
AMAZON.COM
CLOTHES AND HERBS
AMERICANHEALER.WEBSITE
BLACK PEOPLE?
COPS
& Sugar
KD
Chase DuQuesnay Dr. EnQi ReaL

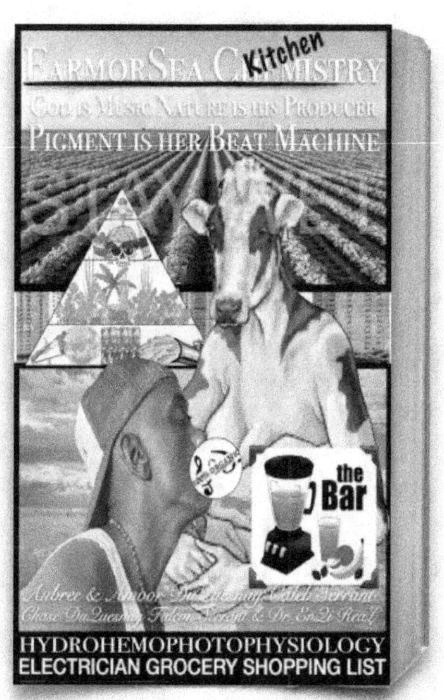
EarmorSea Kitchen Chemistry
God is Music. Nature is his Producer
PIGMENT IS HER BEAT MACHINE
the Bar
Aubree & Armor DuQuesnay Caleb Serrano
Chase DuQuesnay Falcon Forsyth & Dr. En2i Real
HYDROHEMOPHOTOPHYSIOLOGY
ELECTRICIAN GROCERY SHOPPING LIST

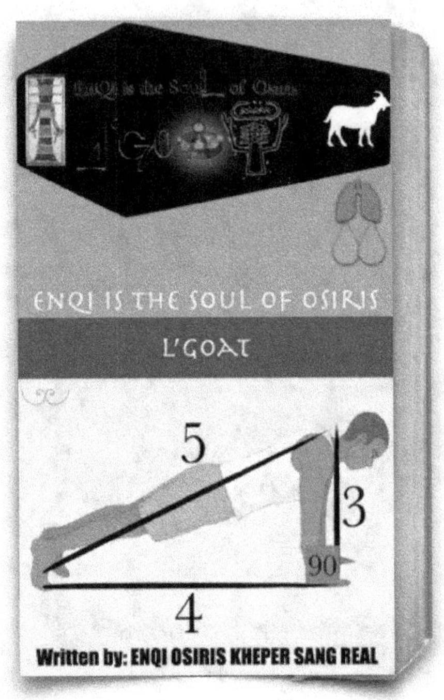

ENQI IS THE SOUL OF OSIRIS
L'GOAT
5
3
90
4
Written by: ENQI OSIRIS KHEPER SANG REAL

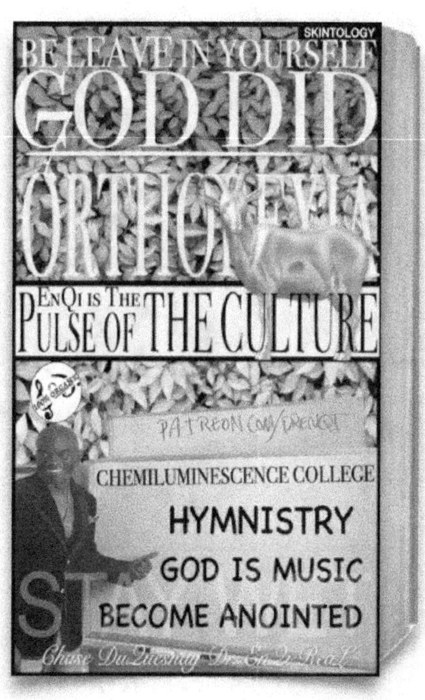
SKINTOLOGY
BE LEAVE IN YOURSELF
GOD DID
ORTHODOXIA
EnQi IS THE
PULSE OF THE CULTURE
100% ORGANIC
PATREON.COM/ENENQI
CHEMILUMINESCENCE COLLEGE
HYMNISTRY
GOD IS MUSIC
BECOME ANOINTED
ST
Chase Du Quesnay Dr. EnQi ReaL

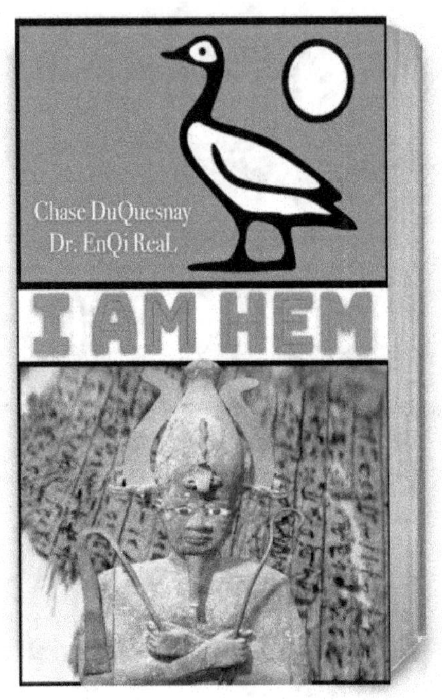

Chase DuQuesnay
Dr. EnQi ReaL
I AM HEM

9 798302 667311